Communicating Health Risks To The Public

Communicating Health Risks To The Public

A Global Perspective

DAWN HILLIER

GOWER

Published by
Gower Publishing Limited
Gower House
Croft Road
Aldershot
Hampshire
GU11 3HR
England

Gower Publishing Company
Suite 420
101 Cherry Street
Burlington
VT 05401-4405
USA

Dawn Hiller has asserted her moral right under the Copyright, Designs and Patents Act, 1988, to be identified as the author of this work.

British Library Cataloguing in Publication Data
Communicating health risks to the public : a global
   perspective
   1. Health risk communication
   I. Hillier, Dawn, 1950–
   614.4'4

ISBN-13: 978-0-566-08672-4
ISBN-10: 0 566 08672 7

Library of Congress Cataloging-in-Publication Data
Communicating health risks to the public : a global perspective /
   edited by Dawn Hillier.
      p. ; cm.
   Includes index.
   ISBN-13: 978-0-566-08672-4 (alk. paper)
   ISBN-10: 0 566 08672 7 (alk. paper)
   1. Health risk communication. 2. Public health--Citizen participation.
  3. Risk communication. I. Hillier, Dawn, 1950–
   [DNLM: 1. Health Education--methods. 2. Communication.
   3. Health Knowledge, Attitudes, Practice. 4. Public Health Administration.
   5. Risk Education Behavior. 6. Risk-Taking. 7. World Health WA 590 C7337 2006]
   RA423.2.C66 2006
   362.1--dc22

2006018467

Printed and bound in Great Britain by TJ International Ltd, Padstow, Cornwall.

Contents

List of Figures

List of Tables

List of Contributors

Woody Caan, Professor of Public Health, Anglia Ruskin University
Woody Caan joined Anglia Ruskin University in 2002 as the first Professor of Public Health, after working as a public health specialist in the UK National Health Service. His special interests are socially excluded young people (for example enabling participation by children with disabilities or promoting mental health in vulnerable adolescents) and health problems related to alcohol (his book *Drink, Drugs and Dependence* was published by Routledge in 2002). He chairs the Social Care Research Group for the NHS R&D Forum and is a member of the national working groups defining Academic Public Health and Health Promotion. His recent publications have mainly related to school health or occupational health. He is an advisor on school health research to the Community Practitioners' and Health Visitors' Association and on the editorial board of the *Journal of Public Mental Health*. He represents voluntary and community sector research on the College of the Academy for Social Sciences.

Lucy Edwards-Jauch, Lecturer, University of Namibia
Lucy Edwards is a Lecturer in the Sociology department of the University of Namibia. She holds an MPhil degree from the University of Cape Town and is currently conducting PhD research on the effects of HIV/AIDS-related adult mortality on family structures in Namibia.

Mary Northrop, Senior Lecturer, Anglia Ruskin University
Mary Northrop is a Senior Lecturer in the Department of Primary Care, Public Health and Sociology. Mary has a background in sociology and has a developing interest in public health risk, particularly the social amplification of risk in relation to obesity.

Shulamit Ramon, Professor of Interprofessional Health and Social Care, Anglia Ruskin University
Shula Ramon is a qualified social worker and Chartered Clinical Psychologist. Her interests are related to psychosocial and policy aspects of mental health; user and carer involvement in research, education, policy planning and partnership working with professionals; social work and political conflict. Shula's research includes the involvement of users as researchers in mental health, evaluation of services and training programmes from the perspectives of users and other stakeholders; action research in mental health which leads to creating better services; promoting wellbeing in the workplace; researching European mental health; evaluation of the involvement of users and carers on the new social work degree; the reactions of Israeli Arab and Jewish social workers to the second Intifada.

Dr Andy Stevens, Principal Lecturer, Anglia Ruskin University
Andy Stevens's main research interests are in disability (especially learning disability) and the history of medicine. He is a long-standing member of the Society for the History of Medicine

and Values into Action. His previous publications were a series of books on disability issues and community care for the Central Council for Education and Training in Social Work (1991–1995) and his doctoral thesis (1998) was an historical analysis of treatment at an institution before and after the NHS implementation. His recent work relates to evaluation of policy and practice in disability services.

Dr Poonam Thapa, Professional Specialist in Gender, Culture and Sexuality

Poonam Thapa is an activist for safer sex. She has worked extensively in South Asia and until 2003 held the position of European Regional Programme Manager for the world's largest voluntary organisation in sexual and reproductive health and rights. She has been a university lecturer in Population and Development and is presently a consultant who brings 25 years of on-ground project experiences from 34 countries in three continents.

Acknowledgements

I would like to acknowledge The Communication Initiative for providing a platform from which to discuss health communication across many countries around the world:

http://forums.comminit.com/index.php?style=1

I would also like to acknowledge the contributions of the following people on the Health and Communication Forum, which commenced on 13 February 2006, on the topic of 'Why Invest in Health Communication?', who contributed to the final chapter of this book:

Nicole West-Hayles, Environmental Health Communication
Paul S. S. Shumba, Consultant
Walter Saba, Senior Program Officer, JHPIEGO – An Affiliate of Johns Hopkins University
James Deane, Managing Director, Strategy, Communication for Social Change Consortium
Ketan Chitnis, Ph.D., Assistant Professor, Manship School of Mass Communication, Louisiana State University, Baton Rouge, LA 70803
Wm. Smith, Executive Vice President, Academy for Educational Development, Washington, D.C.

1 *Introduction*

The World Health Organization (WHO) has identified ten leading risk factors for preventable death and disease worldwide: maternal and child underweight; unsafe sex; high blood pressure; tobacco; alcohol; unsafe water, poor sanitation and hygiene; high cholesterol; indoor smoke from solid fuels; iron deficiency; and high body mass index (BMI), or overweight. WHO hypothesises that 40 per cent of deaths worldwide are due to these ten risk factors alone; global healthy life expectancy could be increased by five to ten years if individuals, communities, health systems and governments took action to reduce these risks by attending to behaviour-change strategies and actions. These actions depend on a complex set of human and societal processes

This chapter provides a broad overview of risk focusing on the various dimensions that affect health risk. These range from consideration of aspects of the risk society, medical-ecology, economics, environmental, socio-political, human-emotional, technological, legal and regulatory (threshold risks), epidemiological mobility to accessibility of health care.

Without risk there is no opportunity for gain

Controversies about risks to public health regularly attract news headlines, whether about food safety, environmental issues, medical interventions, or lifestyle risks such as drinking. To those trying to manage or regulate risks, public reactions sometimes seem bizarre. To the public, the behaviour of those supposedly in charge can seem no less strange. Trust is currently at a premium. Risk has become big business with thousands of consultants providing advice on 'risk assessment', 'risk analysis', 'risk management' and 'risk communication'. The media has become increasingly interested in the subject and terms such as 'risk society' and 'risk perception' regularly grace the pages of newspaper columns and feature on television documentaries and news programmes.

According to Furedi (2002, 5) there are so many apparently expert voices attempting to alert us to new dangers that their advice often seems to conflict and thus confusion reigns over exactly what is safe and what is risky. Safety has become one of the fundamental values of our age. For Furedi (2002, 1), passions that once drove the struggle to change the world (or to keep it the same), are now invested in trying to make sure that we are safe. The label 'safe' gives new meaning to a whole range of human activities, endowing them with unspoken qualities that are meant to merit our automatic approval. For example, 'safe sex' is not just sex practised safely – it implies an entire attitude towards sex and life in general. Moreover, personal safety is a growth industry with hardly a day going by without some new risk to the individual being reported, and another safety measure proposed.

Our inability to come to terms with local, national and global systems failure stems from the fact that television reduces political discourse to sound bites, and academia and medicine organises scientific and intellectual inquiry into narrowly specialised disciplines. As a result we become accustomed to dealing with complex issues, such as smoking, alcohol misuse or obesity, in fragmented components. Yet in the complex world in which we live nearly every aspect of our lives is connected in some way with every other aspect. Consequently, if we limit ourselves to fragmented approaches to dealing with universal health risk issues or natural events, it is not surprising that our solutions prove inadequate. If human beings are to survive the predicaments we have created for ourselves, a capacity for whole-systems thought and action must be developed. Whole-systems thought must include the environment, culture, politics, issues of power and control, institutions and so on.

This book brings together a wide variety of perspectives on risk communication, from the perspectives of health, culture, psychology, entertainment and media. It should be of interest not only to those involved in risk assessment or communication but to anyone interested in the role of science and the media in the political process.

It brings together approaches to risk communication from a number of countries and describes the techniques, including drama, storytelling and scenarios that are used to identify and prioritise key communication issues, and to identify policy responses.

The book also provides a review of the methods and tools available for risk communication and priority setting, which are relevant not only to practitioners but to health planning more generally, and to many other areas of public health and policy formation. The discussion of these techniques is supported by case studies, and is concluded by a chapter reflecting on the conceptual and research issues that still need to be addressed and proposals for different directions in risk communication that keys into the public imagination and gains trust and confidence in the risk messages.

Risks and hazards

Nearly all risk issues involve two hazards: the physical hazard itself (which for the purpose of this book includes risks concerning mental health or rather ill health), and the reaction to it. A lengthy list of examples, from anthrax in the United States mail, mad cow disease in the United Kingdom to SARS in the Far East, demonstrates that elevated fear of a risk is often a larger danger than the hazard itself. At the same time, less concern about a hazard than appropriate can also be dangerous, as is the case with heart disease, sun exposure, food poisoning or motor vehicle crashes. Risk misperception, then, is a hazard, whether the fear is too high, or too low. Take for example the following headline from the *Mail on Sunday* (UK, 8 May 2005):

> At least 12 infected by victim who refuses all treatment
> **TB HUMAN TIMEBOMB**

The medical correspondent Rachel Ellis alerts the general public to the risk to the public from a highly contagious form of tuberculosis (TB) because the authorities, that is the British Government and the medical profession, are powerless to make the individual who is potentially infecting other people accept medical treatment. The article lays the blame firmly at the feet of the Labour Government claiming that it was warned three years ago about the possibility of the TB time bomb in Britain. But it has failed to update Victorian quarantine laws and doctors say they can do nothing to prevent the person concerned passing on the deadly disease because he refuses proper treatment. Ellis claims that the Government now says that it can do nothing because it could breach disease carriers' human rights. Moreover, because of the strict rules on patient confidentiality, the public cannot be warned who the infected person is.

In the context of this book, the aim is not to try to resolve the question of health risk perception or our responses to risk communication, but, in the first instance, to describe an approach or model of causes and consequences of risk communication which seems pertinent to the ethnography of risk communication in different cultures and societies. This lightens the burden somewhat since it would follow, at least from an anthropological perspective with its relativistic suppositions, that ethnography cannot be expected to describe more than an instant, one of the many possibilities, which are engendered by central foundational elements to risk communication as an historical process.

Communicating about risks to public health is of vital importance in many different cultural contexts, quite apart from its importance in government, the health services, local authorities, and the private and voluntary sectors. Because communication needs to be considered at all stages of risk analysis, whether in the village or in post-industrialised cities, it should concern all those dealing with actual or potential public health risks, including individuals, leaders, administrators, medical staff, and scientific and policy advisors.

This book brings two main perspectives to bear. One is that offered by empirical research on reactions to risk. This, for example, explores what influences trust, which types of risk are most likely to be seen as unacceptable or outrageous, how information about probabilities may be understood or misunderstood, and why comparisons between different risks are sometimes misleading. This psycho cultural perspective is extended by considering the wider context – for example the role of the media in determining why some risks rather than others become major public issues or how health risk is or can be communicated through the media. We attempt to understand the privatisation of fault ascribed to certain groups in the context of public health risk, clearly identifying those with responsibility but no choice and those with no responsibility and plenty of choice in their action. We stress the need to guard against taking too narrow a view of the risk issues themselves. We need to understand the socio-cultural context of risk to avoid sending the wrong message, or choosing the right message but failing to convey it.

The second perspective considers risk communication as a decision-making process. Decisions about communication involve much more than just the choice of words and numbers. From this follows the need to consider communication styles and approaches.

Risk and society

For the purposes of this book, four distinct forms of risk are identified: risks that are related to purity, danger and pollution in Mary Douglas's (1966) terms which are essentially locally based and bound up in concepts of spirituality, magic and nature; risks associated with local, technological and environmental dangers (Douglas and Wildavsky 1982). These two forms of risk can be grouped as follows at the level of public policy.

1 Foreign affairs: the risk of foreign attack or encroachment; war; loss of influence, prestige, and power.
2 Crime: internal collapse; failure of law and order; violence and abuse; white collar crime.
3 Pollution: abuse of technology and industry; fears for the environment.

4 Economic failure: loss of prosperity – low paid workers, unemployment; poverty and its
   impact on housing, water supply, waste disposal, transport, education, and so on.
5 Health: disease; accidents, and so on.

The third form of risk relates to socio-cultural risks that are concerned with social capital and
status with a group; and the fourth perspective is concerned with Beck's (1992) notion of
risk, that is, the global exposure of people to risks generated by contemporary industrialised
society, such as nuclear waste. During the modernisation phase, people had willingly accepted
medical and ecological side effects in return for an increase in material welfare, however in
the Western world:

> ... a double process is taking place now. On the one hand, the struggle for one's 'daily bread'
> has lost its urgency as a cardinal problem overshadowing everything else, compared to material
> subsistence in the first half of this century, and to a Third World menaced by hunger. For many
> people problems of 'overweight' take the place of hunger... Parallel to that, the knowledge is
> spreading, that the sources of wealth are 'polluted' by growing 'hazardous side effects'.
>
> (Beck 1992, 20)

These side effects constitute risks and the distribution of these risks is becoming the central
feature of a global society. It is not that the hazards themselves that are necessarily new but the
way in which they are socially constituted are. Consequently, an important defining feature of
risk is its social reflexivity. The risks of which Beck (op. cit.) speaks are primarily generated by
industrialisation, and include threats from toxins, pollutants, radioactivity and nuclear waste,
which may ultimately cause irreversible and invisible damage to the environment.

   The contemporary experience of risk is bound to the concept of reflexive modernisation
and is both scientifically and politically reflexive. Society is intentionally recast as an attempt to
reduce risk but cannot deal with 'the threatening force of modernisation and its globalisation
of doubt' (Beck 1992, 21) because contemporary risks are qualitatively different from the
hazards and dangers experienced in previous periods of history.

> The risks and hazards of today thus differ in an essential way from the superficially similar
> ones in the Middle Ages through the global nature of their threat (people, animals and plants)
> and through their modern causes. They are risks of modernisation. They are a wholesale product
> of industrialisation, and are systematically intensified, as it becomes global.
>
> (Beck 1992, 21)

Risk, for Beck (1992), globalises because it universalises and equalises. It affects every member
of the world population regardless of location and class position. Moreover it respects no
borders. I would argue, however, that global risks do not necessarily equalise since wealthy,
developed industrial countries are in a position to transport their risks, that is, their pollutants
such as toxic waste to less-developed countries. In this way wealthy countries can play down
their own risks while increasing risks elsewhere. Beck further argues that the only possible
solutions to risk, therefore, are supranational solutions such as strategic arms reduction and
international agreements on emission reduction or the proliferation of nuclear weapons.

   From another perspective, one could argue that social institutions not only tend to
standardise ways of life and lifestyle options on a national scale; they are involved in an ever-
intensifying process of globalisation. In individualised societies like the United States or the

United Kingdom, autonomy is always dependent on and restricted by the kind of institutions that give shape to the conditions of social life. On the other hand, this state of affairs makes clear that people have common interests in the quality of the institutions that they so heavily depend on. Exactly because of the penetrative effects of schools, universities, hospitals, social services and industrial companies on the individual life chances of each of us, everyone has a vested interest in the quality of the goods and services that such institutions deliver.

More important is the awareness that local events and personal actions have become heavily dependent on developments and decisions that have their origin in other parts of the world. At the same time, decisions and choices that we make here and now have a serious impact on the life chances of people living far away. For example, each and everyone's adherence to uphold the standards of production and consumption of Western societies not only reinforces the unequal distribution of material welfare and life chances between the rich and poor countries of the world, it also contributes to the continuing exploitation of natural resources that endangers the life and future of coming generations.

Of course, these kinds of global interdependence may be and are ignored on a massive scale in everyday life, but it is no longer possible to deny their existence. That is why, I believe, that we cannot escape from our inherent responsibility for the destiny of other people while acting and choosing in local contexts and on behalf of our personal concerns – even if we do not know these others personally.

Whether one accepts the theories and arguments for global warming, some effects are being felt in parts of the world. For example, climate change has been blamed for vanishing shorelines, decreased crop yields and lower numbers of traditional game, which particularly affects the food supply and way of life for Canada's Far North communities. In the tiny hamlet of Arctic Bay on Baffin Island, Nunavut, researchers have found that changes to the traditional diet are posing an even greater threat to public health.

People were always insecure, but now they are being threatened on a global scale from the risks of pollution and the poisoning of food and water, and the impact of desertification, soil erosion and deforestation that ultimately threaten our health. People's insecurity is also increasingly bound up in the risks of becoming unemployed, and of being deprived of social and physical security. This is the outcome of a worldwide dominance of social institutions that lessen the daily experiences and ethical questions that exceed the limits of their internal criteria and logic. Needs, desires and imaginations that escape their logic are excluded, become objects of discipline, or are suppressed. They are seldom allowed to cause public debates about unforeseen consequences, nor about the ethical dilemmas of modern institutional ways to handle nature (including childbirth), to produce economic growth, or to control the victims of social and economic deprivation.

Nonetheless, Cathy McCormack (1994) created a stir when she declared that the 'let's all go jogging, stop smoking and eat brown bread' type of health promotion campaigns have failed to reduce the health inequalities experienced by people subjected to modern-day poverty. Individualising the problem and the solution only damages the moral and spiritual health of the nation.

> *Modern day poverty is a worse killer than smoking – and it is also passive. That is why people in my community (i.e. Glasgow – EW) are convinced that as much passion must be applied to stubbing out poverty as is being applied to stubbing out smoking. We need homes that are fit to live in and incomes or benefits that prevent us from having to choose between heating and eating.*

> (McCormack 1994, 10)

McCormack (op. cit.) argued that health promotion should be concerned with living conditions because her own living conditions were not on an acceptable level for health. She argued that health promotion campaigns aimed at the individual do not make sense in the absence of adequate living conditions for human beings.

Health as defined by WHO comprises physical, mental *and* social well-being, and as an expression of trust in the present and in the future. Health is both a universal and a specific indicator for people's experience of the quality of their environment and the social relations they share.

Well-being cannot be thought of without referring to trust. If people cannot have trust in themselves, they feel insecure. If they cannot have trust in the sustainability of the environment, they lose perspective on their lives and the lives of their children and future generations. If they cannot have trust in the Government, they feel alienated and excluded from the decision-making regarding their future. Trust is a key category for understanding the construction of societies (Layder 1997). Without trust, societies would tend to be a conglomeration of individuals, more or less ordered to certain interest groups, pursuing their particular interests in competing against each other for the control of resources. Moreover, trust and credibility are central to effective communication about topics of high concern. The key elements in trust and credibility developed by the Center for Risk Communication (2001) are caring and empathy, honesty and openness, commitment and dedication, and competence and expertise.

A changing world

The societal development of industrialised countries, in my view, with which Cosio-Zavala and Gastineau (1997) would sympathise, has led to an almost total elimination of traditional values and belief systems and the roles and functions of their respective institutions. Economic and technological development has simultaneously replaced traditional social systems. Traditions seem to have lost their meanings and functions for societal systems based on the individualisation of social relations in all social sectors and areas. Traditional systems of rationality appear to have been replaced with the rationality of technology. Traditional systems of inter-generational families have, by and large, been replaced with the two-generation family, although a growing proportion of the population lives alone or in single-parent families. Modern societies, therefore, have become post-traditional societies in the sense that they have broken with traditions to a large extent.

Self-realisation and self-sufficiency have now become an overall ideal of human life in modern societies and are the core criteria of success (Romanyshyn and Whalen 1987). Human potential has to be developed to the fullest extent by each individual. In developed societies there is no escape from good advice about how human potential can be achieved. People are subjected to institutions and agencies, which provide an overload of information and advice, resulting frequently in contradictory concepts and measures for improving individual lives. Advice is provided for the selection of the right schools and universities, the purchase of the right clothes, the use of the right language and communication skills, the right foods to eat, the selection of politically correct television channels to watch, the right trust funds to invest in and how to build ecologically sound homes, where to give birth and so on. Whatever people do, there is someone out there telling them how to do it correctly, often supported by some kind of statistical evidence.

Quite apart from governmental bureaucracies regulating public and private life in terms of law and order, developed societies have developed private and public organisations and agencies to design individual life itself. This has led to the development of a considerable industry dealing with every aspect of modern-day life mostly covered up by labels such as 'Do-it-yourself' or 'Self-help'. These labels are euphemisms because the professional advisers or consultants do not really intend people to improve their faculties and skills. Self-help does not mean self-determination, and it certainly does not mean self-organisation or even empowerment of individuals and groups. What the risk communication industry is aiming at is gaining control over individuals and the potential risks they bear for society in terms of development, creativity, solidarity and empowerment through community organisation. The focus is on self and not on help (Romanyshyn and Whalen 1987). It is the self as a discrete unit that is targeted, not the self as a social human being in relation to other human beings. Some would disagree, however, with the gist of the point being made here: those populist books nevertheless encourage people to take control over their own life and to find some mutuality.

The risk communication industry does not deal with communities or social groups but with numbers of discrete units sometimes packaged to target audiences if the issue needs to be transmitted in a relatively short period of time. The relationship between consultant and client is not always characterised by commitment, but by commerce. As soon as people have accepted the advice, that is, as soon as the advice has become the individual's property by making it part of their life, the responsibilities regarding the effects of acting accordingly are theirs. Once the individual starts to jog, the heart failure is theirs. It takes time for the consulting industry to discover whether its advice is sound. Until then, because more and more frequently unequivocal research cannot be delivered, the risks have to be borne by the individual.

Giving advice is an integral part of social relationships because it is an expression of the commitment felt to significant others. This is significant when one considers how health risk is communicated in informal ways between individuals and groups. The difference between this type of advice and the advice provided by the risk communication industry lies in the quality of the relationships between them as illustrated in Table 1.1.

In traditional societies, societal and social processes on the whole are worked through the whole community. In developed societies, these processes are designed by functionaries and experts and are implemented subsequently according to target audiences and target areas. Developed societies have individualised human life by disembedding the individual from their reference groups and treating them as a discrete unit in relation to their social functions

Table 1.1 Quality of relationships in health risk communication

Social relationships:	*Client relationships are:*
• are generally characterised by a strong personal responsibility for individual action	• characterised by the interests of the consultants to lead people on their paths of life
• are characterised by trust	• characterised by efficiency
• have a long-term perspective	• short-term and outcome oriented
• are necessary to build communities and societies through cohesive action	• designed to fix problems
• are based in the context of everyday life	• grounded in artificial settings of professional expertise

(*after* Romanyshyn & Whalen 1987)

(Giddens 1991). Developed societies have sought to organise and impose controls on individual activities but despite the prevalence of a risk communication industry, individuals have been and will be unpredictable in their response to such control mechanisms. This is particularly true with regard to all social areas such as education, health, intimate relationships, entertainment, recreational activities or the entire leisure sector.

Developed societies have undergone major changes in terms of economic policies, technological development, international relations, globalisation and environmental degradation. While considerable wealth has amassed at home, poverty and hunger have increased abroad in so-called developing countries. While excelling in developing and implementing more and more sophisticated technologies at home, almost primitive conditions maintained by extreme poverty prevail in developing countries thus generating increasing numbers of risks not only in those developing countries but also to the developed world as the world becomes increasingly small through globalisation. For as Beck (1999) states, simply by being able to control resources[1], that is global funds, one country is able to control another.

When internal changes in modern societies are investigated, the rapid processes of destruction of traditional values, beliefs, roles and responsibilities, education, families and so on are almost simultaneous with processes of construction of new ways of dealing with the effects of societal changes on a human level. New values and new rituals are superseding old.

Wilde (1994) claims that individuals have a varying 'set point' for risk tolerance. This can be termed 'risk homeostasis'. For some, as the environment gets safer, there is increased risk-seeking (for example, extreme sports). Almost certainly this is true for nations and cultures as well, although risk homeostasis is not a static phenomenon, but one which changes in relation to values, income, perceptions and so on.

Risk in the global village

Risk may be transferred between generations – for example, climate change risk. The Kyoto Protocol is a legally binding agreement between countries to meet emissions reduction targets of all greenhouse gases by 2012 relative to 1990 levels. As of September 2005 a total of 157 countries have ratified the Kyoto agreement (representing over 61 per cent of global emissions). Notable exceptions include the United States and Australia. In March 2001, after reneging on a campaign pledge to regulate carbon dioxide emissions from power plants, President George W. Bush announced his administration's opposition to the Kyoto Protocol.

Risk is also now transferred between nations and regions via trade rules; for example, risks associated with genetically modified organisms (GMO) in food crops are perceived very differently in Europe and some other countries (Japan, Zambia) than they are in North America. Yet the United States, in particular, seeks to demand access to those other markets, using trade rules, regardless of those perceptions.

Knowledge about health risks, and therefore perception and decision-making about potential health risks, may well be more difficult for isolated rural populations than urban populations with access to agencies and the media. The lack of availability of newspapers, radio and television in remote rural areas of the developing world may well restrict access to risk information. This may be further compounded by lack of literacy – reading, health, political

---

1   The US, for example, is highly influential in determining who gets financial aid via the World Bank in line with their foreign policy.

and social – power, influence or funds to take action concerning individual or community health risk decisions.

Structure of the book

This book has been developed to specifically draw on what appears to us to be the key elements that influence the effectiveness of strategies developed to communicate health risks to the public. The conceptual framework for the book involves a number of perspectives ranging from that of the individual standpoint, the cultural context, societal aspects, including the political influences, and the effect of the global village. The authors' interpretations are evident throughout the book and these are captured in the framework from a hermeneutic standpoint.

Moving from global to local and then individual and groups, the book is structured in this way to bring a broad although in no way exhaustive overview of health risk and the context in which health risk communication to the public occurs.

In Chapter 2 the focus turns to the global village. This chapter explores a number of significant global issues pertinent to the study of risk communication. The issues addressed here have been categorised into specific 'globalscapes' concerned with the media and communication, culture, globality and locality, technology, the environment, the exchange of symbols that work to globalise, and the cultural alignments people make within the global village. Contained within these categories are a number of key issues that impact upon individuals and their lifestyles.

In Chapter 3 we begin to explore the cultural meaning of risk. In a world that is increasingly global, with increased migration and communication systems, all societies and cultures are becoming increasingly pluralistic. Moreover, the distance between cultures is diminishing. At the same time, there appears to be an increasing number of cultures and 'imagined communities' emerging with the growth of global diasporas, that are leading to globally-based localisation as well as increasing numbers of localities that are geographically based but not necessarily culturally determined. With increasing specialisation, as a feature of late modernity and globalisation, leading to fragmentation, the question must be: How is the meaning of risk changing around the world in response to globalisation and what consequences do these hold for the communication of risk in contemporary societies? In exploring the context of risk, I attempt to uncover how the balances of power between competing discourses construct, negotiate and control, and in some instances impose, what is accepted as the cultural commonsense of risk in our daily lives in specific environments.

Risk perception is explored in Chapter 4, attempting to understand how people perceive what is risky and what is not. Concepts such as 'magic thinking' in the context of risk come into play. Moving slightly away from the psychology of risk perception to a more societal basis, aspects of the anthropology of risk are brought to bear. This chapter seeks to understand why some risks are ignored and some emphasised and why different groups look at risks in different ways based on an assumption that all risks are moral and politically charged; that all dangers generate blame and culprits, and that culprits are selected in terms of social and cultural frameworks, that assume that:

- risks are culturally biased;
- risks are meaningful;

- perceptions are influenced by socially embedded values and beliefs;
- risk decisions are based on the way of life/worldview of the individual.

Chapter 5 focuses on contrasting styles and approaches to health risk communication, for example: the literary didactic approach appealing to logic; the interactive media that fosters audience participation in television and radio programmes; and online self-assessment of personal risk (health) products are contrasted with, for example, risk communication styles that adopt the storytelling approach using drama, dialogue and acting to generate active participation of audiences, drawing on examples from fieldwork in Africa.

Styles and approaches to risk communication are further explored in Chapter 6 using specific risk concerns, such as communicable diseases, sexual health and obesity, across different groups in different countries as exemplars. In Chapter 7 'Hot cars and cool cigarettes' the effectiveness of risk communication strategies concerned with the temporal resilience of product advertising as cultural icons and the challenge for health and road safety campaigns in changing attitudes and behaviours in young adults is discussed. Andy Stevens looks at media images that reinforce risky behaviours and counter campaigns using both informational and fear appeals.

Reporting on health risks is rarely simple and straightforward. Scientific findings are often complex and ambiguous, and relatively few journalists have special training in science or medicine. Sources of information are often biased, and there is constant pressure to convert dry, technical material into compelling, readable stories, thus news reports are often frightening as well as confusing. Chapter 8 illuminates the tangle of science, politics and economics that often obscures health reporting of mental illness. In this chapter Shula Ramon recounts how the mental health stories are developed and evaluates how the press performed to extract specific lessons and guidelines for identifying and understanding the stories behind the stories that make the news.

In Chapter 9 some exciting examples of alternative approaches for risk communication are explored focusing on popular cultural objects such as soap operas as vehicles for public health risk communication.

In a meeting of the Royal Society for Tropical Medicine, participants heard about one of the most effective interventions for reducing parasitic infestations, a radio soap opera where the plot line included exciting recipes (that is, properly cooked food). The BBC radio soap *The Archers* has inspired a project aimed at improving women's lives in war-ravaged Rwanda. *Urunana*, which translates as 'hand in hand', is designed to provide health information to the public. The drama's storylines are aimed predominantly at women focusing on issues such as contraception, child care, wife-beating and AIDS. Vanessa Whitburn (1999), editor of *The Archers*, claims that a well-constructed soap opera commands a large and loyal audience and is an ideal medium to present life-saving messages in an accessible and understandable way.

The concluding chapter pulls together the potential synthesis of media and cultural studies, which draws upon modelling from anthropology, psychology and population health effects to suggest new directions for effective communication of risk.

2 *View from the Global Village*

This chapter explores a number of significant global issues pertinent to the study of risk communication. The issues addressed here have been categorised into specific 'globalscapes' concerned with globality and locality within the contexts of the media and communication, socio-cultural, technology, the environment, politics and health. We will explore the exchange of symbols that work to globalise, and the cultural alignments people make within the global village. Contained within these categories are a number of key issues that impact upon individuals and their lifestyles.

Whilst each category identifies a specific area for elaboration, it is important to emphasise that they are all interdependent and interactive. Thus it is difficult to entirely separate actions undertaken in one area from its impact on another. As a result, none of the categories have a hierarchical position over any other and therefore are not presented here in an order that represents their importance.

Debate concerning globalisation has fuelled a boom in political, economic, environmental debate and academic publication over the past two decades. The processes that these represent have been in evidence for quite some time than is implied by the manner in which the concept is sometimes used. Some of the dimensions of what is currently described as globalisation have been a feature of many human activities for centuries. These can be discerned, for example, in the excitement, which attended the introduction of technologies in the nineteenth and early twentieth centuries, including the telegraph, telephone, radio, photography and film. The globalisation process today is marked by the accelerated pace at which informational and cultural exchanges take place, and by the scale and complexity of these exchanges (on the latter, see Appadurai 1990, 6). These include the volume and increasingly international flavour of the goods that are available to the public, international tourism and migration, internationalisation of ownership of property and businesses, shared possession and use of media products and icons across national boundaries. The global availability of an increasing range of moving images in films and television programmes, press and magazine articles, photography and music is difficult to ignore.

Facilitated by the new technologies, it is the sheer speed, extent and volume of these exchanges and their effect on everyday life that have engaged popular imagination. Such technologies range from electronic mail to the satellite dish, and although these are clearly not accessible to all, they have obviously been directly or indirectly responsible for exposing many different sorts of people to new influences. Such technologies are able to uncouple culture from its territorial base so that, detached and unanchored, it travels across the world to all those with the means to receive it. The accelerating effects of electronic communication and rapid transportation that can move people from one location to another create a structural effect that McLuhan (1964, 185) called 'implosion'. By this he meant the bringing together in one place all the aspects of experience where one can simultaneously sense and touch events and objects that are great distances apart. The centre-margin structure of industrial civilisation disappears in the face of global synchronised and instantaneous experience. In what has become an evocative and iconic formulation, McLuhan asserted that 'This is the New World of the global village' (1964, 93). But global space is not in any way similar to a tribal village.

The debates about globalisation cross many disciplines. For example, Giddens (1990) firmly situated globalisation as a consequence of modernity, whose dynamics radically transform social relations across time and space. More specifically, he argued that globalisation occurs in four key domains: the extension of the nation-state system; the global reach of the capitalist economy coupled with the international division of labour; and a global system of military alliances. Robertson (1992) anchors the development of globalisation in an earlier history and outlines a five-phase model in which many more institutions, actors and ideological and cultural elements play a role. Hannerz (1990) argued that the assumption common to much globalisation discourse, as did theories of cultural and media imperialism before it, that globalisation and its cultures move from the 'centre' (that is, modern North and West) towards the periphery in largely one-way flows was erroneous. He argued that centre-periphery relations are much more complex; cultural flows can and do move in multiple directions. This tension is reflected in the many contributions on globalisation. The central question is whether there can be a global society. Such a development would be more than just the sum of the parts (global economic relations, global political institutions and a shared globalised culture); it would be based around new forms of identification.

The globalised world it is argued can be defined by a single word – *integration* – and all the threats and opportunities in this globalised world flow from integration and it is symbolised by a virtual object – the *World Wide Web* – which could potentially unite everyone. Friedman (1999) considers that we no longer have a first world, second world or third world. There is just a fast world and a slow world. The globalisation system is a dynamic, ongoing process that involves the inexorable integration of markets, nation-states, and technologies to a degree never seen before. This is happening in a way that is enabling individuals, corporations, and nation-states to reach around the world farther, faster, deeper and cheaper than ever before. People are either in the fast world or in the slow world. Friedman equates globalisation to running in the hundred-metre sprint run over and over and over again, and no matter how many times you win, you have to race again the next day. If you lose by one tenth of a second, it is as if you lose by two hours – the gap is so wide that it is also producing a powerful backlash from those brutalised or left behind by this new system.

The increasing interdependence of national economies – as well as increasing social and cultural global linkages – means that economic fluctuations and their social impacts now reverberate on a global level. Growing poverty and insecurity are linked to social conflict, extremism, violence, crime, child labour and other social problems. Because the source of these problems involves a global dimension, their solutions cannot be found only on the local level: local and national action must be complemented by action taken at the global level.

For Waters (1995), the contemporary accelerated pace of globalisation is directly attributable to the explosion in signs and symbols. Human society is globalising to the extent that human relationships and institutions can be converted from experience to information; to the extent it is arranged in space around consumption of symbols rather than the production of material goods, that value-commitments are badges of identity; to the extent that politics is the pursuit of lifestyle, and that organisational constraints and political surveillance are displaced in favour of reflexive self-examination. These and other cultural forces have become so overwhelming that they have breached the banks not only of national value-systems but also of industrial organisations and political-territorial arrangements. Globalisation does not imply, however, that every part of the world has become Westernised and capitalist; rather, that social, economic and political arrangements in every sector must establish their position in relation to the capitalist West.

For Friedman (1999, 1) the globalised system is built around three overlapping and interacting balances: the nation-state (that is the *superpower*), the multinational companies or *supermarkets*, and, in Friedman's terms, the relatively unrecognised *super-empowered individual*.

The first is the traditional balance between nation-states. In the globalised system, the United States is currently the dominant superpower and all other nations are subordinate to it to one degree or another. The balance of power between the United States and the other states is still important for the stability of this system. The second balance in the globalisation system is between nation-states and global markets. These global markets comprise investors moving money around the world by the click of a mouse. Friedman refers to them as 'the electronic herd'. This herd gathers in key global financial centres, such as Wall Street, Hong Kong, London and Frankfurt, which he calls 'the supermarkets'. The attitudes and actions of the electronic herd and the supermarkets can have a significant impact on nation-states today, even to the point of triggering the downfall of governments.

The United States is the dominant player in maintaining the globalisation 'gameboard' (Friedman, 1999, 2). But it is not alone in influencing the moves on that gameboard, sometimes pieces are moved around by the obvious hand of the superpower, and sometimes the invisible hands of the supermarkets move them around.

The third balance in the globalisation system is the balance between individuals and nation-states. Since globalisation has eliminated many of the boundaries that restricted the movement and reach of people, and because it has simultaneously networked the world, it gives more power to individuals to influence both markets and nation-states than at any other time in history. Consequently, there are now not only superpowers and supermarkets, but also super-empowered individuals able to act directly on the world stage without the traditional mediation of governments, corporations or any other public or private institutions. For example, Jodie Williams who won the Nobel Peace Prize in 1997 for her contribution to the International Ban on Landmines achieved that ban not only without much government help, but also in the face of opposition from the Big Five major powers. Her secret weapon for organising 1000 different human-rights and arms-control groups on six continents was simply 'E-mail' (Friedman 1999, 13).

Nation-states, and the American superpower in particular, are still hugely important today, but so too now are supermarkets and super-empowered individuals. To understand the globalisation system, it is vital to 'see it as a complex interaction between all three of these actors: states bumping up against states, states bumping up against supermarkets, and supermarkets and states bumping up against super-empowered individuals' (Friedman 1999, 13). Significantly, all these players are concerned to a large extent with risk, whether financial, political or social and indeed health. Management of risk communication is of paramount importance in the global village to the extent that information and misinformation can be transported around the world very quickly.

Symbolic exchanges in the global village

Waters (1995) argued that globalisation resulted primarily from the exchange of symbols. For him, globalisation proceeds much more rapidly in contexts in which relationships are mediated through symbols and rituals. Economic globalisation is therefore most advanced in the financial markets that are mediated by monetary tokens and to the extent that production is dematerialised. Political globalisation has advanced to the extent that there is an appreciation of common global values and problems rather than commitments to material interests. However, material and power exchanges are rapidly becoming displaced by symbolic exchanges, that is, by relationships based on values, preferences and tastes rather than by material inequality and constraint. In the context of this argument, globalisation might be seen as an aspect of the progressive 'culturalisation' of social life (Waters 1995, 124). An example of this is evident in the following story brought to our attention by BBC News:

US 'harming' Uganda's Aids battle (BBC 2005)

The UN's special envoy on fighting Aids in Africa Stephen Lewis has accused the United States of endangering the gains Uganda has made in containing the disease. Lewis told the BBC that Uganda – under pressure from Washington – was putting greater emphasis on abstinence to tackle the disease than condoms. His remarks follow a report by US health campaigners saying the country was facing a condom shortage. Uganda, however, denies any change in policy and the US has rejected the UN accusation.

Mr Lewis said: 'Over the last eight to 10 months, there's been a very significant decline in the use of condoms, significantly orchestrated by the policies of government. At the moment, the government of Uganda appears to be under the influence of the American policy through the presidential initiative of emphasising abstinence far and away over condoms,' he said.

He suggested US President George Bush, who launched his multi-billion dollar campaign to tackle Aids in Africa two years ago, was acting under the influence of the religious right in the US. A senior US official rejected Mr Lewis's criticism, saying the current administration supported condom use as part of a balanced programme that included prevention.

Source: BBC NEWS published 30 August 2005.

Although condoms are themselves a Western concept and product, to withdraw or delay in the delivery of condoms to Africa, with the aim of changing a country's cultural approach to something as basic as sexual activity, could be considered a real misuse of power. Moreover, in the following case study by Lucy Edwards (Lecturer in Sociology of Gender at the University of Namibia) effectively illustrates the point that globalisation of fundamental Christian ideals, such as abstinence and being faithful, is not a simple or easy task in different cultural contexts.

Case Study: HIV and the ABC: A duel between Western-Christian morality and African patriarchy

To date, governments, donor agencies and non-governmental organisations have mounted massive HIV/AIDS awareness campaigns in a bid to stem the increase in infection rates. The central prevention message has been abstinence, monogamy (be faithful) and condom use under the rubric of the ABC rule. Empirical evidence suggests that out of the ABC mantra advocated in prevention campaigns, condom use is the most effective prevention method.

Attempts to de-emphasise condom use in favour of abstinence and monogamy will increase women's vulnerability to HIV exposure. Empirical studies show that Western-Christian constructions of sexuality as encapsulated in ABC prevention models do not reflect the majority experience. These models put forward abstinence, monogamy and condom-use as the rational decisions individuals ought to make to practice safe sex. It is hoped that the positive results the ABC rule yielded in Uganda can be replicated elsewhere. This is not always the case. To understand why one may have to look beyond Western Christian sexual morality. More particularly one would also have to look at how gender and class intersect with socio-cultural constructions of sexuality.

Sexuality and by extension HIV/AIDS cannot be abstracted from its structural base. A number of anthropological and sexual-cultural studies in Namibia indicate that the ABC rule overlooks the complex social, economic and cultural roots of prevailing sexual cultures. Empirical evidence further suggests that the ABC rule is an over-simplification of very complex sets of social power relationships that overshadow sexuality.

KNOWLEDGE, AWARENESS AND BEHAVIOURAL CHANGE

Our findings confirm the results of Demographic and Health Surveys namely, in countries with high levels of HIV prevalence there are also high levels of AIDS awareness. Despite high levels of knowledge about modes of HIV/AIDS transmission, modes of prevention, and the impact of HIV/AIDS, infection rates are still increasing in some demographic groups, particularly amongst young women in the 15–24 year age group (UNICEF 2005). This disjuncture between knowledge and sexual behaviour modification debunks rational choice theories about sexuality that assume complete individual autonomy over sexual and reproductive decisions.

ABSTINENCE BEFORE MARRIAGE

AIDS campaigns promote abstinence before marriage however in Namibia, only 29 per cent of the adult population are currently in formal sexual unions. Of these, 19 per cent have marriage certificates and a further 7 per cent are in stable consensual relationships without having gone through a legal or traditional marriage. Some 56 per cent of adults have never been married. This indicates a decrease in formal marriage compared with the 1991 Population Census statistics.

The concept of marriage is often loosely applied and based on a continuum that ranges between formal marriage to temporary and intermittent cohabitation. The boundary between stable union and casual sexual relationship is also quite fluid. There is a diversity of sexual unions brought about by a number of historical, social-economic and cultural factors like polygamy, labour migration, urbanisation, economic dislocation, monetisation, violence and mass poverty.

If stable unions could be defined as marriage or cohabitation then the minority of sexual relationships occur inside stable unions. In our study over 70 per cent of those who are sexually active were not in a stable union. The link between sex and marriage forged in HIV/AIDS campaigns ignores the socio-cultural construction of sexuality and the centrality of sexuality in the construction of gender identities. Manhood is often associated with virility and sexual conquest. Most respondents in our study thought that abstinence was unrealistic in practice. Men reported societal and peer pressure to prove manhood by being sexually active.

Women reported a lack of sexual autonomy to make decisions about abstinence due to unequal gender power relationships and economic exigencies. Widespread gender-based violence diminishes women's ability to autonomous decision-making about their own bodies. In addition, violence creates fear and silence. Married women in polygamous relationships have been identified as a high-risk group. Despite legal protections they are not able to abstain from sex. Culturally, sex is regarded as a husband's right and a wife's duty.

The decline in formal marriage, the introduction of wage labour and the monetised economy have led to the economic dislocation of single women who migrate to urban centres, seek male patronage and use sex as a survival strategy.

BE FAITHFUL AND POLYGAMOUS SEXUAL CULTURES

The decline in formal polygamous marriages did not end polygamous sexual cultures. Often it is assumed that people in non-permanent relationships are more at risk of HIV exposure, but the polygamous sexual cultures also make women in stable unions a high-risk group. Despite their own monogamy, women in stable unions are not much safer than single unmarried women due to male promiscuity. A SADC study revealed that HIV infection rates are six times higher among married women than among single women (Tibinyane 2003).

Adultery has historically been something that only happens to men. When one man had sexual relations with the wife of another man, then adultery was committed against the male spouse of the woman involved in the adulterous affair and not against the female spouse(s) of the man who had the adulterous affair (Becker 1995). This places the notion of faithfulness in a very particular cultural and historical context.

Although in decline there are groups who still uphold wife lending and husband lending. The practice of okujepisa/oupanga makes it socially acceptable for a husband to lend his wife to a male friend or person of high social status to strengthen the male friendship (Talavera 2002).

The reverse is also acceptable when a wife invites her husband to sleep with her female guest (ibid.). Some cultures still practice wife inheritance (levirate), where a man may inherit a deceased brother's wife. This poses a risk if the brother died of HIV/AIDS-related causes (ibid.).

Our empirical results point to widespread non-monogamous sexual cultures that result in diverse and complicated sexual networks. Many women accept or are forced to accept multi-partner sexual relationships despite the risks. There is a cultural and socio-economic basis for multi-partner sexual relationships. It is legitimated by culture and tradition. In addition, social and economic changes add to the complex structure of society as new classes begin to form. The new social groups that are coming into being are urban wage earners, informal sector traders, working and non-working poor and urban elites who by virtue of their privileged positions in politics, the administrative system or business have considerable incomes. High-income males from privileged positions often become the sugar daddies to young girls and the partners of women in transactional sexual relationships.

There are different factors that result in male and female promiscuity. Past studies have linked HIV/AIDS to male sexual promiscuity (Le Beau et al. 1999), but with economic displacement women are increasingly forced into multi-partner sexual relationships as a means of securing a livelihood. This increases the rate of change in sexual partnerships and size of sexual networks.

The Christian morality of monogamous marriage is central to the 'be faithful' aspect of the ABC rule. In a number of countries in Africa this constitutes less than half of all sexual unions. Most sexual relations occur in the context of the polygamous family (United Nations

2002a). Most Namibian cultures practised some form of polygamy. Only with Christianisation did monogamy present itself as a sexual norm.

Polygamy has been an integral part of traditional social organisation. It had important social and economic functions in the traditional pastoralist and subsistence economies (Becker 1995) where it contributed towards male material wealth and social status. Women's lack of ownership and control over productive assets allowed men to control women's sexuality, fertility and labour (ibid.). In most societies only the male head of a polygamous family could acquire land from the chief. He then allocated land use to his wives. In many of the subsistence farming communities, female access to productive land is still predicated upon her relationship with a male relative, particularly a husband. Land reform programmes have not touched customary land tenure patterns. This could be one way of redressing the structural imbalances that make women vulnerable to HIV exposure.

CONDOM USE

Of the three elements of the ABC rule condom use is the most practised prevention strategy. However, condom use is still subject to male preference. Patriarchal power relations and economic dependency often make it impossible for women to negotiate condom use.

Culturally women are taught to show a passive disinterested aloofness in sex to confirm male sexual dominance in relation to female innocence and ignorance (Becker 1995). Widespread gender-based violence creates a culture of fear that inhibits women's sexual expression.

Fertility desires play a role in condom use. Decisions about fertility are often not matters of personal choice, but made to meet family and social-cultural obligations (United Nations Secretariat 2002a). Fertility desires often outweigh health considerations, be it in relation to HIV exposure or the possibility of mother-to-child transmission (ibid.) Fertility desires are still central to the construction of masculine and feminine identities. Fatherhood is often synonymous with manhood and motherhood synonymous with womanhood. In some cultures men who have not procreated are excluded from community-level decision-making. This creates pressure to prove fertility through unprotected sex (McFadden 1992).

In African literature and other cultural forms, African womanhood is exalted by motherhood, and women's humanity is recognised in relation to their fertility. Some Namibian languages do not distinguish between womanhood and motherhood since they are regarded as synonymous.

There is further speculation that women may want to prove their fertility and thereby good health, to hide their HIV-positive status in the fear of abandonment or stigmatisation (United Nations Secretariat 2002b). In general, condom use is inconsistent and situational (Epinge 2003). People will only use condoms at the beginning stages of the relationship, but will stop after a while without being certain of the partner's HIV status and sexual behaviour (ibid.).

CONCLUSIONS

HIV/AIDS campaign messages have been too generic. There should be greater segmentation of risk groups to allow for targeted campaigning that address the particular circumstances of different risk groups.

The ABC rule may apply to some. It may, however, be unrealistic for those who rely on sex for their physical survival, those who are in extremely unequal sexual power relationships and those who are subjected to sexual violence. We should also address the structural basis of inequality and vulnerability. Prevention campaigns have been silent about polygamous sexual cultures and the economic exclusion that create a high-risk environment for HIV exposure. Awareness campaigns have elevated the Christian monogamous marriage to the most desirable norm but it is not the only or most common form of sexual union.

The baseline survey results point to relatively high levels of condom use, but given the complexity and multiplicity of sexual networks, situational condom use still poses risks. The challenge lies in promoting increased and consistent condom use.

There are also particular high-risk groups with little bargaining power to negotiate condom use. These include women in stable unions where polygamy and other forms of non-monogamous sex are practised as well as women who enter into transactional sexual relations or who use sex as a means of securing a livelihood.

The challenge lies in providing women with safe sex options they can control such as the female condom or other female-initiated prevention methods (for example microbicides). Religious and ideological doctrines that reject condom use deny some vulnerable groups the only possibility of protection.

The concept of globalisation is an obvious object, claimed Waters (1995, 3) for ideological suspicion because, like modernisation, a predecessor and related concept, it appears to justify the spread of Western culture and of capitalist society by suggesting that there are forces beyond human control that are transforming the world. This book makes no attempt to hide the fact that the current phase of globalisation as it impacts on risk perception and risk communication is precisely associated with these developments. Globalisation is the direct consequence of the expansion of European and American culture across the planet via settlement, colonisation and cultural imitation. This is clearly exhibited in the field of health care and lifestyle.

HealthScapes: impact and relevance of global organisational policies

As the chief executive of the Royal Society for the Promotion of Health, Professor Richard Parish said (2004 – private communication) 'Health is determined to a large extent by the way in which we organise our societies, and by the policies and priorities that countries adopt. Health is a function of the environmental circumstances we create and the lifestyles we encourage. The health services are undoubtedly important, but they form only one part of the complex jigsaw that determines health in the world of the twenty-first century. In a very real sense, the state of our health is determined by the health of our State.' This is graphically described in the examples from Anne-Christine D'Adesky's book *Moving Mountains: The Race to Treat Global AIDS* (2004). She describes the current situation, for instance, where, as Haiti's poverty has increased, so too have crime, violence, prostitution and the illegal drug industry. With its economy at standstill, due in part to the international embargo, the Government has been unable to do much in the battle against HIV. Mexico, too, is a society that has considerable challenges, with the largest population than any other metropolis, reflecting the very rapid growth of a city that cannot keep pace with the demands for housing, water, education and health services. In the post 9/11 period, as the United States has tightened control of its borders to Mexico, poverty has increased, tourist dollars have reduced and unemployment is high. Sex work and drug trafficking are increasing – two factors that are contributing to the continued spread of HIV, particularly among women.

D'Adesky (ibid.) demonstrates very clearly the global interconnection between countries and how financial sanctions imposed by the United States and the World Trade Organization's alignment with 'big pharma' have acted to impede the treatment of HIV in developing countries. There is a serious lack of access to affordable AIDS medicines for not only poor people in wealthy countries such as the United States, but also for the developing world. The huge gap in access has allowed people in the developing world to die while rich people in rich countries survive. Poverty is the connecting thread between both rich and poor countries, which also links AIDS to other diseases of the poor such as tuberculosis, and in Africa and Asia, malaria and sleeping sickness.

EnvironScapes: health risk and the environment

Another important aspect of the interconnectedness in the global village concerns the environment. There is evidence that we are experiencing accelerating social and environmental disintegration in nearly every country of the world, as revealed by increases in poverty, unemployment, inequality, violent crime, failing families and environmental degradation. These problems stem in part from a massive increase in economic output over the past 50 years that has forced demands on the ecosystem beyond that which the planet is capable of sustaining. The continued drive for economic growth as the organising principle of public policy is accelerating the breakdown of the ecosystem's regenerative capacities.

Although exposures to environmental risks contribute significantly to the burden of disease among children and adolescents (Smith et al. 1999, WHO 2002), there are still gaps in our knowledge about the magnitude and regional distribution of the environmental burden of disease (EBD) among the young. For the WHO European Region in particular, there are no estimates.

Climate change, for example, whether one accepts the doomsayer's or the sceptic's arguments or not, is impacting not only on the lives of individuals in one country but worldwide. Take for example the effects of one of the more recent hurricanes – Katrina in September 2005:

> *Of the approximately 16 000 people living with HIV/AIDS in Louisiana, 12 849 resided in communities most affected by Hurricane Katrina, including nearly 7400 in the New Orleans metropolitan area alone. Many displaced or otherwise affected by the disaster are seeking care and treatment services elsewhere in the state or in other states, compounding the challenges due to the hurricane itself.*
> Kaiser Network Interview with Louisiana State AIDS Director, 26 September 2005

MediaScapes

In my travels around the globe it seemed to me that Western culture has penetrated even the most remote areas. This appears to be mainly through a process of media communication. When visiting a remote village in Ghana I saw a young child wearing a tee shirt proclaiming Coca-Cola to be the 'best'. On questioning the level of understanding of the meaning of the advertisement, the child revealed that Coca-Cola was delivered to the local store. This local store was a wooden, one-room shack on the side of the road in the village.

The emergence of large international media companies which own media interests in numerous countries increasingly function to undermine any sense of a national media tied to a particular nation-state. Their interests are global and they have done much to generate international markets rather than national markets for their products, particularly promoting new technologies such as satellite, which have no national boundaries. They have benefited from the general deregulation and the marketisation of modern culture in the last two decades. There has been a continuing 'mediatisation' of culture (see Brunn and Leinback 1991). Against such obvious power of these companies, it is a relatively simple matter to hypothesise the weakness of individual consumers. It seems uncontroversial to suggest that the effect will be to produce mass consumers of the products of such companies on a world scale.

Patterns of social interaction and information flows are increasingly occurring across national boundaries to form new bases of social, political and cultural identity. Communication networks, previously responsible for vertical integration of a society, are stimulating emerging patterns of social interaction, political organisation, changing ideological assumptions and cultural forms as well as information flows, transitionally in a process of horizontal integration and articulation.

Once a country makes the leap into the system of globalisation, its elites begin to internalise this perspective of integration, and will always try to locate themselves in a global context. Unlike the Cold War system, globalisation has its own dominant culture, which is why it tends to be homogenising. In previous eras this sort of cultural homogenisation happened on a regional scale. Friedman (ibid., 8) gives the examples of the Turkification of Central Asia, North Africa, Europe and the Middle East by the Ottomans or the Russification of Eastern and Central Europe and parts of Eurasia under the Soviets. Culturally speaking, in his view, globalisation is largely, though not entirely, the spread of Americanism.

Globalisation is also characterised by its own demographic pattern exemplified by the rapid acceleration of the movement of people from rural areas and agricultural lifestyles to urban areas and urban lifestyles that are more intimately associated with global consumerist trends in fashion, music, food, and entertainment. Along with these lifestyle trends, the risk-taking and risk-seeking behaviour becomes central to the value system of the urbanites. These include smoking, gambling, high alcohol consumption and increasingly hedonistic risk. By hedonistic risk I am referring to those risks associated with amateur extreme sports, binge drinking, the Ibiza phenomenon, where large numbers of young people holiday with the express purpose of drinking, dancing, taking drugs and having multiple sexual encounters. Paul Lewis's (1999) explanation below for this is an exemplar of the nature of globalisation:

In the mid to late 1980's Ibiza played an important role in the burgeoning 'dance' music scene. A new type of music that had started out in the nightclubs of Chicago was filtering through the sound systems of the developing clubs in the resorts on the island of Ibiza. An important catalyst in the success of these clubs was the emergence at the same time, of the drug Ecstasy (MDMA). These two elements combined to attract young people to the island to experience the hedonistic, marathon dance parties that were developing a Europe-wide reputation for the island.

In 1987 two UK DJ's visited the island (Paul Oakenfold and Danny Rampling) and liking the scene that they experienced there, decided to import it to the UK club scene. Before long a similar underground dance music scene had developed in the UK and with this there was a huge shift in youth culture.

With the massive growth and diversification of the UK rave/dance music scene through the late Eighties and early Nineties, so the scene in Ibiza developed apace. In the eyes of UK and European clubbers, Ibiza was seen as the place where it all began, a sort of 'holy grail' of clubbing and hedonism. With its widening reputation and with the crossover of the underground dance music scene into the mainstream (witness the rise of the 'brand label' clubs in the UK – Ministry of Sound, Cream, Club UK and similar examples in Ibiza such as Manumission), Ibiza has become a place of the mainstream, and thus gained huge popularity ...

(Lewis 1999)

An unidentified man in the United States reported having sex with multiple partners while under the influence of the club drug methamphetamine, also known as crystal meth. It is theorised that amphetamines may suppress the immune system, allowing the HIV virus to replicate more quickly in the body. Methamphetamine also contributes to unsafe sex practices that make the spread of HIV more likely. This highly addictive drug releases people from their inhibitions, leading otherwise sexually responsible men, women and teenagers to engage in risky sexual behaviour.

(Healthology staff 2005)

Conclusion

Waters (1995) takes the three arenas of the economy, polity and culture to be structurally independent. The argument, however, does make the assumption that the relative effectiveness of the arenas can vary across history and geography. A set of arrangements, perceived to be more effective in one arena can penetrate and modify arrangements in the others just as a more effective set of arrangements in one country can penetrate and modify arrangements in another. Changes in the practice and rituals surrounding risk are one example of this, the research by Lucy Edwards above is another.

These themes can now be linked to an argument about the creation of the global village. Waters argued that the types of exchange that predominate establish the link between social organisation and territoriality in social relationships at any particular moment. Different types of exchanges in his view apply to each of the arenas indicated above. Respectively these are:

- material exchanges including trade, tenancy, wage-labour, fee-for-service and capital accumulation;
- political exchanges of support, security, coercion, authority, force, surveillance, legitimacy and obedience;
- symbolic exchanges by means of oral communication, publication, performance, teaching, oratory, ritual, display, entertainment, propaganda, advertisement, public demonstration, data accumulation and transfer (research), exhibition and spectacle.

For Waters (1995, 9) each of these exchanges exhibits a particular relationship to location, respectively.

- Material exchanges tend to tie social relationships to localities: the production of exchangeable items involves local concentrations of labour, capital and raw materials; commodities are costly to transport which militates against long-distance trade unless there are significant cost advantages; wage-labour involves face-to-face supervision; service delivery is also most often face-to-face. Material exchanges are therefore rooted in localised markets, factories and shops. Specialist intermediaries (merchants, sailors, financiers and so on) who stand outside the central relationship of the economy are required to carry out long-distance trade.

- Political exchanges tend to tie relationships to extended territories. They are specifically directed towards controlling the population that occupies a territory and harnessing its resources in the direction of territorial integrity or expansion. Political exchanges therefore culminate in the establishment of territorial boundaries that are coterminous with nation-state societies. The exchanges between these units, known as international relations (that is, war and diplomacy), tend to confirm their territorial sovereignty.
- Symbolic exchanges liberate relationships from spatial referents. Symbols can be produced anywhere and at any time and there are relatively few resource constraints on their production and reproduction. Moreover they are easily transportable. Importantly, because they frequently seek to appeal to human fundamentals they can also claim universal significance.

It follows that the globalisation of human society is contingent on the extent to which cultural arrangements are effective relative to economic and political arrangements. Waters expects the economy and the polity to be globalised to the extent that they are culturalised, that is, to the extent that the exchanges that take place within them are accomplished symbolically. We would also expect that the degree of globalisation is greater in the cultural arena than either of the other two.

In the context of risk, the fact that modern people trust their societies and their lives to be guided by expertise, does not necessarily mean that they leave all risk decision-making to others. Modern people engage in monitoring activities because they are aware of risk. People do constantly observe, inquire about and consider the validity of expertise. Modern society is therefore for Giddens (1990) reflexive in character. Social activity is constantly informed by flows of information and analysis that subject it to continuous revision and thereby constitute and reproduce it. 'Knowing what to do' in modern society, even in such traditional contexts as kinship, childbirth and lifestyle risk, almost always involves acquiring knowledge about how it is done from books, television programmes or experts in the specialist field, rather than relying on experience of self and others or the authoritarian knowledge of elders.

The particular difficulties faced by modern people are that this knowledge is constantly and rapidly changing so that living in a modern society appears to be uncontrolled or chaotic. The proliferation of knowledge and symbols promotes two kinds of reflexivity. It promotes a pattern of what Lash and Urry (1994) refer to as 'reflexive accumulation', the individualised self-monitoring of production and of expertise and an accompanying increase and widespread tendency to question authority and expertise.

It promotes an aesthetic or expressive reflexivity in which individuals constantly reference self-presentation in relation to a normalised set of possible meanings given in the increasing flow of symbols. People monitor their own images and deliberately alter them. These images may fall into four different cultural types which will be explored in the next chapter.

3 *Cultural Meaning of Risk*

A stranger in a strange land would hardly expect to communicate effectively with the natives without knowing something about their language and culture. Yet, risk assessors, managers and communicators have often tried to communicate with the public under the assumption that they and the public share a common conceptual and cultural heritage in the domain of risk. That assumption is false and has led to failures of communication and conflicts (Slovic 2000, 189).

A growing number of authors have commented that people in late modernity are constantly faced with risks as phenomena that must be negotiated so that we may live a 'reasoned' and 'civilized' life (see for example, Giddens 1991, Beck 1992, Douglas 1992, Lash et al 1996). For Beck (1992, 87), the contemporary focus on risk is part of what he terms 'a social surge of individualization' in which people have become compelled to make themselves the central focus of how life is lived and where hazards, dangers, threats or crises are frequently seen as individual problems rather than socially based.

Risk concepts, however, have emerged out of Western cultures and predominantly those experts identifying, categorising, analysing and communicating about health risk are from Western societies and cultures, imbued with their values and beliefs. If the people who need to be mobilised for implementation of the reduction of health risk, are in most cases from different cultures, whose perceptions of illness, health, health care and health problems are based on local traditional concepts and minimally influenced by concepts of modern medicine, the risk communication process will be considerable, without any real evidence that it will ultimately make a difference to mortality or morbidity.

In this chapter we will explore the cultural meaning of risk to attempt to clarify the contextual meaning of culture used as a basis for understanding health risk communication.

The cultural debate

Culture has been studied and defined in many ways by multiple scholars representing various disciplines. It is not our intention to provide and exhaustive account of the debates around culture, however, Adler (1997, 15) provides a useful starting point for a basis for the exploration of culture in the context of health risk communication. She has synthesized many definitions of culture and says that culture is:

- Something that is shared by all or almost all members of (a) social group.
- Something that the older members of the group try to pass on to the younger members.
- Something (as in the case of morals, laws and customs) that shapes behaviour, or ... structures one's perception of the world.

Culture is more than the arts: it is a framework for our lives. It affects our values, attitudes and behaviour. On the one hand we are actors in our culture and we each have an effect upon it while on the other we are shaped by our culture. According to Levo-Henriksson (1994), culture covers the everyday way of life as well as myths and value systems of society. Roos (1985) sees culture as a system of lifestyles and as a common dominator for lifestyles. Kroeber and Kluckhohn, however, who in 1952 categorised 164 separate definitions of culture, formulated their own definition:

> *Culture consists of patterns, explicit and implicit, of behaviour acquired and transmitted by symbols, constituting the distinctive achievement of human groups, including their embodiment in artefacts; the essential core of culture consists of traditional (i.e. historically derived and selected) ideas and especially their attached values; culture systems may, on the one hand, be considered as products of action, on the other, as conditional elements of future action.*

(Kroeber & Kluckhohn 1952, 181; cited by Adler 1997: 14)

Culture for me though is a much more dynamic and complex phenomenon that also carries our strongest feelings concerning change, stress, danger, fear and protection across time and between generations. This becomes relevant when we begin to consider how and why people respond to the 'softer' aspects of risk communication, that is, through storytelling in various forms.

According to Adler (1997, 15–16), culture, values, attitudes and behaviours in a society influence each other. Values can be defined as factors that are explicitly or implicitly desirable and that affect our decisions. Our values, which do not need to be conscious, are based on our culture. Our attitudes express our values and trigger us to act or to react in a certain way toward something. Attitudes are always present when people act even if they do not see them. The behaviour of individuals and groups in turn influence the society's culture.

Adler (1997) gives six dimensions that can be used to analyze cultural differences. She pays attention to the understanding of the nature of people; a person's relationship to the external environment; the person's relationship to other people; the primary mode of the activity; people's orientation to space; and the person's temporal orientation. All of this affects the ways in which we respond to health risk communication.

Risk and cultural types

According to Douglas (1992, 18) and Thompson (1992, 182–198) there are four distinctive ways of organising modern society. These four cultures, as Douglas terms them, are each in conflict with the others. People tend to embody one of the cultures and play out a lifestyle that exemplifies that cultural type as illustrated in the following descriptions expounded by Thompson (1992).

INDIVIDUALISTIC OR ENTREPRENEURIAL LIFESTYLE: CHARACTERISTIC – DEVELOPMENTAL

Those subscribing to this cultural type tend to be characterised as 'Driving in the fast lane'. They tend to be entrepreneurial, competitive with wide-flung, open ego-focused networks of people. They enjoy high-tech instruments and generally lead a risky lifestyle, insisting on the freedom to change commitments. Persons who subscribe to this cultural lifestyle are on the whole knowledgeable, enthusiastic and fashion conscious (even to the most fashionable way of giving birth or engaging in extreme sports). Individualist's philosophy of life and cultural bias embraces politics, aesthetics, religion, morals, friendships, food and hygiene. They have a cosmopolitan, neophiliac and wide-ranging consumption style. For them, nature is benign and they view resources as being abundant.

The individualist perception of time is that short term dominates long term and they have a preference for laissez-faire governance. Their commitment to the organisation only lasts as long as it is profitable to the individual. The individualist cultural alignment is based on a way of life that is free to bid and bargain and needs nature and people to be robust to refute arguments of those who are against any action they have in mind. If things go wrong, either the unproductive individual or the external distortions of the market gets the blame. Individualists fear anything that would impair the functioning of the market, such as war.

HIERARCHICAL LIFESTYLE: CHARACTERISTIC – ORGANISATIONAL

Hierarchists are understood to benefit from a type of lifestyle which formally adheres to the customs and values of the institutional establishment and its time-honoured traditions. They insist on maintaining a defined network of family and friends (driving in the slow lane). They view their knowledge as almost complete and organised. For them nature is robust, but only within limits. This lifestyle justifies the hierarchist's control of nature and the environment through the institution of regulations and procedures on the individualist's projects. Their solution to 'pollution' (and here pollution can also be understood as deviation from the expected norm of society) is to change nature or people to conform to society (this is most clearly manifested in population control strategies).

The hierarchist consumption style is essentially traditional with strong links to the past and others within the group. The hierarchist favours high-tech virtuosity on a large scale and is biased toward ritualism and sacrifice in order to maintain control. They view resources as scarce and prefer bureaucratisation through increasing transaction costs. For them the greatest risk lies in the loss of control (that is, public trust). Their commitment to institutions takes the form of correct procedures and discriminated statuses that are supported for their own sake. Their watchword is 'loyalty'. People within this lifestyle need structure, however, if things go wrong, the 'victim' gets the blame; the present outcry about obesity is a prime example of this. Hierarchists want well-established rules and procedures to regulate risks. Hierarchists fear crime, delinquency, and other risks that would disrupt the careful ordering of society.

ENCLAVIST OR EGALITARIAN LIFESTYLE: CHARACTERISTIC – HOLISM

Egalitarians are characterized by their commitments towards a lifestyle comprising social institutions which esteem the values and ideals of redistributive justice and a safe and secure environment.

They are against formality, pomp and artifice. They reject authoritarian institutions, preferring simplicity, frankness, intimate friendships and spiritual values. Nature and people are ephemeral, fragile and pollution (either physical or spiritual) can be lethal. Their knowledge is viewed as imperfect but holistic. This lifestyle is entered in fundamental disagreement with the policies of the development entrepreneurs (individualist) and with the organising hierarchists, and with the fatalism of the isolate. They see resources as depleting and lean towards a frugal and environmentally benign approach to technology and industry.

They consider that society needs to conform to nature; consequently, their cultural bias favours fundamentalism (not necessarily in a religious sense) and millenarianism (a belief in a future period of ideal peace and happiness). Their preferred economic theory verges on Buddhist and thermo-dynamic approaches to economics. For them the long-term concerns dominate short-term activities and gains. The egalitarian views the risks associated with global development strategies as catastrophic, irreversible and inequitable. Their commitment to institutions takes the form of collective moral fervour and affirmation of shared opposition to the outside world. Their watchword is 'voice'. People in this lifestyle need to be activists and if things go wrong, the system gets the blame. Egalitarians focus on low-probability but catastrophic risks such as nuclear power, because fear of disaster keeps members in line.

ISOLATE OR FATALIST LIFESTYLE: CHARACTERISTIC – FATALISM

Fatalists or isolates are characterised by a feeling of lack of control over the world. They are identified as those socially isolated individuals who, while living outside the other three groups, are disposed to adopt a cultural attitude which rationalizes their perceived inability to influence the course of events in the world (Dake, 1991). Their preferred lifestyle is characterised as eclectic, withdrawn but unpredictable, with a refusal to be recruited to any cause. Friends do not impose upon the isolate, and they are not hassled by competition or burdened by obligatory gifts, nor irritated by tight arrangements or timetables. In this cultural type, nature and people are seen as unpredictable and capricious.

They take a fatalistic approach to life and view the acquisition of resources as a lottery. The scope of knowledge is irrelevant and learning is a matter of luck. Their priority is to cope with the chaos of daily life; the survival of the individual is the paramount concern, and thus they devise short-term responses to cope with erratic mismatches of needs and resources. Their consumption style is isolated; traditionalist but they have weak connections to the past or others. The isolate often has low productivity but is highly innovative. If things go wrong, 'it's the poor that gets the blame'. People in this lifestyle are marginalised through structural imbalance. They need to maintain their dignity through acceptance of their situation. Fatalists do not bother fearing risks, as they do not think they can prevent them – rather, they hope to simply be able to roll with the punches.

Douglas (1992), believes that each individual buys into a lifestyle that best exemplifies their personal values and beliefs about the social, cultural, environmental, political and financial world. To understand the way in which our social experience affects how we think we need to recognise two distinct ways in which society may exert pressure on an individual. Douglas (1992, 9) uses the term 'grid' to refer to restrictions that arise from the system of social classification, for example, the distinction between lord and commoner or between man and woman. Grid refers to the internal structuring of a society and, in this sense, is the set of rules, which govern individuals in their personal interactions. Strong or high grid means strongly defined roles, which provide a script for individual interaction. Towards the weak end of this axis, the public signals of rank and status fade and ambiguity enters the relationships. Individuals no longer have the guidance of a script, but are valued as individuals and relate to each other as such. The constraints become correspondingly weaker, until they take only the generalised form of respect for each person as a unique individual.

Douglas (ibid.) uses the term 'group' (the strength of the boundaries set between insiders and outsiders) to refer to the extent to which an individual's interactions are confined within a specific group of people who form a sub-group within the larger community. Where the group is strong, there is a clear boundary between members and non-members. Membership confers benefits and though it may be possible for an individual to leave the group, that will have high costs. For example, membership of the medical fraternity confers valued benefits, which include financial as well as social support. However, being excluded from the group (such as losing one's license to practice) can leave the individual exposed and vulnerable. However, members of the group are able to exert considerable pressure on the individual to conform to its requirements; examples of this can be found in some youth culture where serious consumption of alcohol on a Friday night is vital among young men. Even the type of drink is defined – strong lager or beer, for example. This goes hand in hand with violence and aggression when the group is threatened. Members participate to show solidarity and group loyalty.

By contrast, where the group is weak, the individual is free to form relationships or negotiate exchanges with anyone, and the resulting network of interactions constitutes a myriad of overlapping groups, with sub-groups of individuals who interact only with themselves. Of course, individuals can and do belong to a number of different sub-groups at the same time, but one is generally not a member of the Labour Party while being a member of the Conservative Party since their ideals allegedly clash. People can and do move between groups as they change their allegiances based on new information and changed beliefs.

High-grid and high-group organisations or cultures are hierarchical in nature and conform closely to group norms and responses to risk, placing their trust in institutions. This aligns itself to the techno-scientific formulations of risk where risk is a largely taken-for-granted objective phenomenon. The focus of research is the identification of risks, mapping their causal effects, building predictive models of risk relations and people's response to various types of risk. Studies, mainly in the fields of science, engineering, psychology, economics, medicine and epidemiology, are undertaken adopting a rationalistic approach which assumes that expert scientific measurement and calculation is the most appropriate standpoint from which to proceed. This demands the adoption of a realist approach to risk and to an extent, ignoring the socio-cultural context in which the risk arises.

In contrast, low-group and low-grid organisations are highly individualistic, preferring a self-regulatory approach to risk. While such structuralist models of risk responses may be criticized for their rigidity, they do begin to offer a view on risk that goes beyond a focus on the individual and their psychological or cognitive response to risk to an interest in the socio-cultural context in which individuals exist and through which they make judgements about risk.

Douglas and Wlidavsky (1982) identified several types of social organisation that *selected* different hazards as particularly relevant, specifically listing war and crime as unacceptable risks for hierarchic/bureaucratic societies (high-grid, high-group), economic collapse for market/individualist societies (low-grid, low-group), and environmental pollution for egalitarian/sectarian societies (low-grid, high-group).

Risk and culture: symbolic communication

There is a growing awareness that risk is a social and cultural concept and that risk perceptions depend less on the nature of the hazard than on the political, social, and cultural contexts in which they take place. Normally, a group's memory of risk and danger consists of individually held memories that influence people to interact in particular ways. These interactions produce the complex group dynamics that make up the social environment and culture of a group

– be it an organisation, a subculture or a community. These dynamics change when the group undergoes the stress of a change or some sort of shock. This is because people's memories store stresses and shocks differently than normal memories.

These memories are imprinted more deeply into our minds, in a different system in the brain. They do more than influence; they *compel* people to interact in certain ways that create predictable interpersonal dynamics which are often played out in the rituals of a group. For example, in the Akan tribe in Ghana, a woman will generally hide her pregnancy for as long as possible fearing that knowledge of her pregnancy will attract the evil eye or bad luck. Thereafter, the baby is not named (except for the name of the day on which it was born, for example Adowa for Monday born) for some weeks following birth as the risk of death is high and the child is regarded as a visitor. During this period recently delivered women wear a traditional blue and white cloth depicting their status. Once the period of waiting is over, there is a naming ceremony. The mother wears gold cloth and there is a big celebration – a kind of 'coming out' into society ritual.

In another example, a teenage girl in the UK attended a family planning clinic to get the morning-after pill. This was not her first visit. When questioned by the practitioner about the background to why she had unprotected sex, she explained that 'condoms were for wimps' (that is, cowards). There is a similar case study in Tulloch and Lupton (1997, 4) in which a young, female, black, working-class girl who had been in and out of remand homes, commented that 'condoms are chicken', again meaning cowardly. In her world, as in the world of the British teenager, where risk is an everyday occurrence, where her group stole cars and drove them fast, where they smoked pot and where they knocked over old women for their handbags, risk is deeply embedded in their culture, in its economics as well as its leisure activities. For young people like this, who enjoy stealing, fast cars and taking illegal substances, using condoms might well seem wimpish or chicken.

Douglas (1966; 1992) and later, Lash (1993; 2000) both highlight the importance of risk cultures and of shared notions of risk within cultures and communities. For Douglas, risk perceptions and risk choices are highly symbolic, delineating the boundaries between self and other. For Lash, they are aesthetic understandings and judgements, mediated through lifestyles and membership of social groups. So, for example, Paulo's behaviour and perceptions of what it means to smoke and drink, to use drugs or to have unsafe sex will bear far more relation to what is considered normal or cool, within his reference group, than it will to any external calculation of risk.

Bourdieu (1986; 1990), however, is concerned both with the individuality of actions and their embeddedness in cultural and structural contexts. In hierarchical social spaces, young people have different economic and cultural capital resources, and differential access to the 'rules of the game' of lifestyle and choice. Their choices may be understood in terms of 'habitus' a concept defined by Pierre Bourdieu which includes the person's beliefs and temperament and prefigures everything that that person may choose to do. These choices are not limitless (indeed all possible choices are unknowable to the individual and therefore are not options). Thus, the concept of habitus challenges the concept of free will, for in normal social situations a person relies upon a large store of scripts and a large store of knowledge, which present that person with a certain picture of the world and how they think to behave within it.

Moreover, a person's habitus cannot be fully known to the individual, as it exists largely within the realm of the unconscious and includes things as visceral as body movements and postures, and it also includes the most basic aspects of thought and knowledge about the world, including the habitus itself. Consequently, Paulo's choices are indeed his own, but are steered by his life experiences, the culture and contexts he lives in and the capital he accrues; they are unique to him, but they may also be shared. Evans (2002), putting forward the related concept of 'bounded agency', expresses a similar view:

> Young people are social actors in a social landscape. How they perceive the horizons depends on where they stand in the landscape and where their journey takes them. Where they go depends on the pathways they perceive, choose, stumble across or clear for themselves, the terrain and the elements they encounter. Their progress depends on how well they are equipped, the help they can call on when they need it, whether they go alone or together and who their fellow travellers are. If policies and interventions are to be made effective, we need to sharpen our awareness of the interplay of structural forces and individual's attempts to control their lives.
>
> (Evans 2002, 265)

Risk and ritual

For Le Bretton (2004, 3–5) adolescents do not have the same fatal, irreversible vision of death that their elders do. Each has a tendency to feel that they are special, different from others, outside the common law. Death is still a vague notion in their eyes and they feel it cannot affect them – it only affects other people. In parallel, they test it; play with it like a dangerous partner that may grant self-esteem to those who confront it with open eyes. Paradoxically, this inflation of the ego is also based on an inner need to show others that they can react fearlessly. The fear of losing face or the need always to show a specific skill is a major source of risk-taking.

Van Gennep (1960 edition) captures this experience in his description of a rite of passage where individuals experience liminality. A liminal phase is equated to limbo where initiates are neither a part of the social group they came from (childhood) nor a part of the group to which they are being initiated (adulthood). In the pre-liminal phase, initiates are seen to ritually die so as to leave their old life. The final phase is a post-liminal one where a few successful individuals celebrate their membership of the new social group and all that it entails. Douglas (1966) and Turner's (1969) concept of ritual to generally indicate stereotyped actions that remain faithful to an established cultural pattern can perhaps begin to offer an explanation of the cultural dynamics of the ritualised processes of youthful risk taking. Their invariability grants them their efficacy in different domains, ranging from promoting the restoration or creation of social solidarity and order, to effecting changes of status, or to taking risks for themselves or others. Moreover, it is precisely through this changeless nature that rites play an important role in complementing the information provided by mythology in this context. Its link to the mythology of youth is so close that it can be said that rites are the enactment of myths.

Rites are commonly divided into two kinds: public and private. The first is concerned with social groups that are beyond the level of the individual, family or domestic units, friends or gangs. The settings for risk rituals are often villages, compounds, schools or hospitals, public houses, streets and even supermarket car parks after dark. One informant recalled the following story about a group of fourteen- and fifteen-year-old girls who used to meet in the local supermarket car park in a small town in south-eastern England every evening.

The boys were about thirteen – well who'd want to talk to them? One or two were older but they were nerds. We'd stand on our side and they would stand on their side and we'd shout across – teasing you know … we never went any closer. They were skateboarding mostly and making a lot of noise – you know – taking up lots of space. Then one day the car park was locked – fences all around and we couldn't get in – the sign said it was being done up or something. So we had to find somewhere else to go. Laura said that some guys hung out at the other supermarket car park and perhaps we should go there. So we did. There was a gang of older boys – smoking and drinking something. They came over and asked if we'd like a drink – so we did. Trudy went off with one boy to the corner and later the others paired off and I was left … so I went home. It wasn't as much fun. Trudy and Annie got pregnant and I know one of the other girls had an abortion.

Changing the cultural dynamics of the groups initiated the girls into the rituals surrounding teenage smoking, alcohol consumption and sexual experimentation. These increased and compounded both the girls' social and health risks (if they refused to comply with the norm, that is, engaging in smoking and so on), and risks to their safety (if they rejected the encouragement of the older boys to engage in alcohol consumption or sexual activity).

The second group of rituals are more to do with the individual or family. Rituals have several phases (see van Gennep 1960; Turner 1969), which alternate between liminal and structured periods. This means that apart from the symbols that surround rites one also examines their sequence. Moreover, since the actions take place in particular areas and among people who have some kind of relationship, spatial referents and social relationships also provide important information. Through them one can obtain information about conceptions of space and time and about patterns of social interaction.

The cultivation of fear

Fear, according to Furedi (2005), is fast becoming a caricature of itself. It is no longer simply an emotion or a response to the perception of threat. It has become a cultural idiom through which we signal a sense of unease about our place in the world. Moreover, popular culture encourages an expansive, alarmist imagination through providing the public with a steady diet of fearful programmes about impending calamities – man-made and natural.

Furthermore, Furedi (2002) postulates that safety has become the fundamental value of our times. He argues that passions that were once devoted to a struggle to change the world (or keep it the same) are now devoted to trying to ensure that we are safe. Furedi believes that the word 'safe' gives new meaning to a wide range of human activities, endowing them with qualities that are meant to gain our immediate approval. Safe sex is not just sex practised healthily – it implies an entire attitude towards life (as discussed by Poonam Thapa in Chapter 6). The safe-drinking campaigns express a moral statement about life. Personal safety is a growth industry which started in the United States but quickly crossed the Atlantic to the United Kingdom, where hardly a day goes by without some new risk being reported and another new safety measure being proposed. Nowhere is this seen more than in the response to childhood risk in modern societies.

The culture of risk-aversion goes far deeper than the over-the-top regulation. The phenomenon that Frank Furedi has termed 'paranoid parenting' has become an orthodoxy that governs every aspect of child-rearing. This parenting extends beyond the actual parent to the Government playing the parental role. This consciousness about the vulnerability of children and the notion that society should organise itself around protecting them from any potential harm is not about consciously avoiding risk. It is about redefining the ordinary features of everyday life as problematic. Perhaps driven by media scare stories and parental anxieties, the culture of risk aversion comes from the very top of society.

It is UK Government policy to highlight the dangers posed to children by everyday parental behaviour, schooling experience and social interaction. Stay safe (which includes safety from maltreatment, neglect and abuse, violence and sexual exploitation; safety from accidental injury and death; safety from bullying and discrimination; safety from crime and antisocial behaviour; having security, stability and being cared for); be healthy (which includes physical and mental health, sexual health, healthy lifestyles and avoiding illicit drugs), enjoy and achieve, make a positive contribution and achieve economic well-being are prominent targets for the official attempts to show that 'Every child matters' (HM Government 2004).

Running through all this is the assumption that children are at risk from the people around them, and particularly those closest to them; and that what society needs is a code of conduct to ensure that the safety and self-esteem of the child are paramount, to be placed above all other considerations. In such a climate, no wonder parents become paranoid – to resist the orthodoxy invites the label of child abuser (Halpin 2005).

What drives this culture is not concern about children but adults' fears. The decline of adult solidarity and the increase in suspicion and mistrust govern the relationships between adults engaged in the task of child-rearing, making an already anxious situation even more troubled. This generates a broader loss of faith in people's ability to make a difference to society at large, and the belief that any attempt to make a difference risks making things worse. The focus of adult activity narrows to the minutiae of child-rearing, and the focus of child-rearing becomes protecting children from the world of risks that surround them, rather than initiating them into adult society.

National difference in risk behaviour

National differences in risk behaviour stem from two sources: differences in long-standing cultural values and interpretations or differences in current situational circumstances. Differences in individualism – collectivism and uncertainty avoidance, for example, identified by Triandis (1989) as important dimensions of cultural variation, reflect national differences in typical responses to certain types of situations that are mediated by long-standing differences in cultural values. While it is true that the goals and behaviours advocated by a culture evolved – at some point in the culture's past – as adaptive reactions to persisting situational circumstances, cultural values also take on a life of their own and become an independent influence on the behaviour of members of that culture (Schwartz 1992).

However, situational differences in countries' current political and economic environment also contribute to observed national differences in behaviour. If, for example, risk or uncertainty is associated with smaller rewards in one country than in another, then rational self-interest would predict national variation in risk-taking. Thus, national differences on some behaviour are not easily and conclusively attributable to one or the other of these two sources. McDaniels and Gregory (1991) have voiced concern that many researchers fail to distinguish between these two classes of explanations. That is, observed national differences are often treated as cultural in origin, without any attempt to distinguish between cultural versus situational determinants. More than in other research domains, conclusive insights in cross-cultural research require a combination of methods and approaches. It is important to know – but difficult to establish – whether observed national differences in behaviour are truly cultural, that is, are the result of long-standing differences in cultural norms and values which are not easily modified, or whether they are more malleable and transient because they result from current situational circumstances.

The ability to predict national differences in degree of risk-taking, for example, is of considerable practical importance in the arena of cross-cultural risk communication, since differences in risk attitudes offer the door to the creation of integrative health communication solutions, for instance, solutions that leave both sides better off than if they had the same risk attitude.

Conclusion

Culture is more than the arts; it is a framework to our lives. It affects our values, attitudes and behaviour. Risks, for Mary Douglas (1992) are embedded in a complex system of beliefs, values and ideas. People perceive risks through different 'frames' that reflect their world views and concept of social order. These frameworks can influence definitions of risk, allocation of responsibility and blame, evaluations of scientific evidence, and ideas about appropriate decision-making authority. The automatic, unconscious processes of groups and cultures are more powerful than logic, good intentions or social rules. This is especially true under conditions of stress, threat or trauma. On the one hand we are actors in our culture and affect it and on the other we are shaped by our culture. Communicating risk in the context of culture and cultural differences demands an even more complex set of algorithms to formulate appropriate risk communication approaches and transmit appropriate risk messages. Understanding how individuals perceive is the next part of this complex jigsaw concerning communicating health risks to the public and is explored in the following chapter.

4 How Do We Perceive Risks?
by Woody Caan and Dawn Hillier

Santee, California, 6 March 2001

Suspect, 15, Had Made Repeated Threats Before Attack Near San Diego (LA Times)

Carrying a black revolver and wearing an enigmatic smile, a diminutive 15-year-old boy opened fire on the campus of a suburban San Diego high school Monday morning, killing two students and injuring 13 other people.

St. Paul, Minnesota, 6 March 2001

5-Year Olds Suspended for Having Gun in School (Star Tribune)

Two 5-year-old girls were suspended from Hayden Heights Elementary School in St. Paul after one of them brought a loaded gun to school in a small handbag.

Philadelphia, Pennsylvania, 5 March 2001

8-Year Old Brought Gun to School (Las Vegas Sun)

'He said he's going to shoot me. He said he's going to make it a blood bath and throw me in the Dumpster,' Fatimah Edwards, 9, told WCAU-TV. She reported the threat to a teacher, who called police.

On 5 October 2003 psycho-illusionist Derren Brown put a gun to his temple and shot himself five times in the head in a game of Russian roulette on live television (UK Channel 4)[1]. More than three million people watched the mind control expert undertake his illusion, which was performed outside of the UK to avoid tight gun laws. Outrage and criticism ricocheted around the globe but despite criticism by senior police, there were fewer than 100 complaints made to Channel 4. 'What sort of person wants to put the bullet in the gun which might kill Derren Brown? ... some 12 000 people applied ...' (*The Guardian*, London). It seems that it does not take much of a dare to make many people do really hazardous things.

---

1 www.derrenbrown.co.uk/news/roulette (viewed January 2005).

Picture this scenario

There are five drunken teenage boys milling around after school in Amarillo, Texas[2]. One of them carries a gun 'for self protection'. He takes the gun out of his pocket and boasts that he has played Russian roulette. The others boys do not know what this is but suggest that they play the game. The boy with the gun – who has not played Russian roulette in reality – agrees and puts one bullet in the chamber of the gun.

- If you were one of the parents of these boys how would you perceive the risk and how would you transmit the risk to your son?
- If you were a school counsellor or welfare officer, how would you understand the risk and how would you communicate the risk to the boys?
- If you were one of the boys and felt uncomfortable about playing this game, how would you interpret the risk and what would you say, if anything, to your friends?

Most young people are happily integrated into their society, but there are groups of teenagers who are on the fringe, finding it hard to find meaning in their lives or perceive themselves in positive terms (Le Bretton 2004, 1). Le Bretton believes that risk-taking particularly affects this age group. The reasons for putting their lives in jeopardy in order to exist are numerous and complex. Dares, attempted suicides, drug taking, eating disorders and reckless driving are common ways in which adolescents jeopardise their existence. Abandonment and either family indifference or overprotection may be the root cause of such acts.

According to Kopel (2000) more than 135 000 children carry a gun to school every day. While these figures are contested Kopel agrees that there is a serious problem and that the fault lies not with gun ownership but with other antecedent factors, such as drug use. He claims that since drugs are readily available in the inner city, despite extremely severe national prohibition, it is foolish to expect that gun controls will take guns out of the inner cities.

In terms of risk perception parents do not want any harm to come to their children and would assess the danger in absolute terms – that one of them will die as a result of this game. The counsellor or welfare officer will take into account the general pattern of teenage behaviour. The young person themselves may either relish an experience that could leave battle scars to be proud of if they survive, or may feel trapped in a situation that they recognise as highly dangerous but they cannot lose face before their friends. The question is what, to these adolescents, is acceptable versus unacceptable violence? Young people's perception of that boundary is where past bullying plays a significant part. That, in turn, may be the trigger that makes teenagers carry guns and shoot at other students in their schools.

In a questionnaire study by Newman et al (2005) students who reported having been bullied, verbally abused, isolated and unpopular in high school were more likely to view the use of a gun, for example, as a reasonable means of settling a score. They were prone to sympathise with the violent, often lethal, actions of bullied victims in the questionnaires' scenarios. Children seem to experience an accelerated development of antagonistic behaviour if they have been exposed to ongoing stress at certain periods in their development. Moreover, Newman et al (2005) suggest that the effects of environmental and social stressors during an isolated period of development have the potential to be lasting.

---

2   Texas gun laws again received a 'D-' because its laws are among the worst in the country at protecting children from gun violence. In 2002, the most recent year for which data is available, 222 children and teenagers in Texas died from gunfire. (www.bradycampaign.org/facts/reportcards/2004/tx.pdf).

Adolescent narcissism generates a paradoxical feeling of invulnerability and frailty. Elkind (1967) calls this specific self-image a 'personal fable', which is common in adolescence and can sometimes lead adolescents to endanger their life, persuaded that they can cope with the situation and that the frailties of others do not affect them. This feeling is ideal for triggering actions which can potentially cause considerable harm. Playing games involving risk nourishes their confidence in their own resources, whereas everyday life often causes acute awareness that reality seems to slip through their fingers. Attitudes such as recognising the need for security, or weighing up decisions and actions, and searching for information are rarer among young people than adults.

Adolescents are far more attracted by the gratification of their peers and narcissistic restoration, wanting to prove that 'they can do it' and so the awareness of danger often eludes them.

We're doomed, Captain Mainwaring!

Private Frazer's catchphrase from the long-running BBC comedy *Dad's Army* (www.bbc.co.uk/comedy/guide/articles/d/dadsarmy_7771975.shtml) resonates with generations of British audiences. Statistically, British society has never been safer, but the political commentator Joan Bakewell (2006) summarises a preoccupation with sudden, horrific death from external causes: 'The vast majority of us die in our beds. So why do we have such a distorted sense of risk?'

There is already a considerable research literature concerning risk perception. It is therefore, not the intention in this chapter to present an exhaustive account, but rather to identify aspects of risk perception that are important in communication.

'Risk' has become a highly topical term during the past two decades. Risks related to technological developments, working conditions, residential settings, lifestyle activities, public health, environmental hazards, global ecological changes and so on attract substantial publicity and are widely discussed in society. Salient examples include both high-frequency non-catastrophic events (for example exposure to electro-magnetic fields from mobile phones, power lines and microwave cookers) and the low-frequency but catastrophic events (for example a nuclear power station rupturing). Consider consumption of sweet fizzy drinks, which increases the probability of clinical obesity. This is a very common behaviour and the issue in risk perception is how to evaluate something so mundane. Many of us do not make risk decisions about nuclear reactors but we do make decisions about how we drive and maintain our cars and daily activities like eating, drinking, and whether to take the bus or walk to work.

Risk can be conceived as either a potential for harm or as a social construction for worry

Some hazards that society takes for granted are actually catastrophic for those people exposed; for example in a head on collision between two cars travelling at 60 miles per hour, there is a high probability that everyone in the vehicles will be killed. Even if there is a survivor, there is a high probability of brain damage that will restrict their lives for the rest of their lifetime. One of the most difficult challenges in the area of health risk is that in poor societies contracting HIV is a catastrophic event, currently experienced by millions of people.

Perception is sometimes dulled and sometimes exaggerated. Sometimes our perception of risk is inappropriately, actively manipulated and distorted; for example, benzodiazepine drugs which can be very useful in some circumstances, are now with hindsight acknowledged to have been overused in a variety of inappropriate and hazardous cases (Ashton 1986, 2004; Lader 1987, 1991). Both natural and man-made disasters create a heightened awareness of dangers to humankind. They can stimulate rapid mobilisation of resources; for example in 2005 a new and hugely expensive tsunami early warning system for the Far East developed from cooperation across countries. In contrast, everyday dangers like AIDS that affect millions of people seem incapable of producing international action, for example, at the G8 summit in 2005.

For many people, the problem of taking risks is not the objective level of danger (the way an insurance company keeps actuary figures of risk) but an emotional one (Douglas and Wildavsky 1982). For example, according to work undertaken for the Driver and Vehicle Licensing Agency (DVLA), the most persistently dangerous drivers are those who believe they are particularly safe drivers (perhaps that they have just missed out on being racing drivers). The Formula One racing car driver Juan-Manuel Fangio was once asked by an interviewer whether he drove very fast on the public highway. He replied, 'Absolutely not. I always worry that coming round the next corner will be a driver who thinks he is Fangio.' The drivers (mostly aged under 25) in the DVLA study had actually experienced multiple accidents and yet did not perceive their driving as high risk: the objective evidence of their series of car crashes was not the most important factor.

The perception of risk depends on the context. If you were playing football in a club it would not be as dangerous as playing football on a minefield. So, with the schoolboy gun scenario, the parents have to work on the context – they need to reduce the frequency of their sons becoming drunk and out of control and vet the friends they are involved with. They will never be able to control the specific risk incident but can do work upstream to prevent the event. The counsellor or welfare officer needs to persuade the boy with the gun to not carry the gun all the time. In the incident situation, the boy cannot stop his friend carrying a gun but he may persuade the other boys to delay the game by using a *delay* (don't act on impulse) – *distract* (changing people's immediate attention to something else) – and *divert* technique. However, they are all much more likely to get seriously injured when they have a pattern of getting drunk.

Politicians, health practitioners and policy makers tend to treat risks as calculable and technical. Therefore, they approach risk communication from the basis that if people were informed and understood these calculations, then their behaviour would change. But for many people, lay and professional alike, the problem is that they do understand the risk. Take, for instance, doctors and nurses who smoke: they understand the hazards very well, but the risks are outweighed by their perception of the benefits smoking brings. They know the consequences for other people and are well able to make risk calculations, but when it comes to themselves, they cannot apply these calculations to themselves. For them, 'If I am a player in the game, the probabilities shift in my favour' and this is an example of 'magical thinking'. The odds of winning a big prize on the lottery are approximately 14 million to one – but the advertising says, 'It could be you.' People who play the lottery habitually, when they become personally involved believe that the probability of winning a big prize shifts in their direction.

If such magical thinking is applied to many situations and risks, it is associated with outcomes like pathological gambling. The person who sees themselves as a stud may be aware of sexually transmitted infections but cannot emotionally accept that it could happen to them. This type of perceived invulnerability happens in every country and to both sexes. For example, one undergraduate student who believed he was 'God's gift to women' used to put on his lucky socks every weekend, around which he had built up a complex mythology which increased his confidence, before going out to score with a new woman. The simultaneous emotional context ensured that he would be both lucky in love and invulnerable to any consequences such as the gonorrhoea that was rife at the time. This was an educated student of economics, not someone who was incapable of understanding risk. But he could not apply such calculations to his own behaviour.

If interventions are planned to alter people's perception of risk, they will only work if they are appropriate to the emotional state of the person receiving the intervention. In the 'cycle of change' model (Prochaska and de Clemente 1982) some interventions need to be timed for contemplative periods when the target is open to considering change. A few interventions seem to work best in highly charged emotional situations such as a driver's first arrest for drink driving (for example Court Diversional Schemes under probation) or, in the drugs field, when a heroin user first discovers she is pregnant. These are the exception. There are very few occasions when you would try to shift perceptions of risk in such highly charged states and even then, interventions do not work for everybody.

It is much more common to attempt interventions in more relaxed and happy circumstances, such as using a home visit around a child's first birthday party to review accident prevention in the home setting. Nutritional advice is best linked to happy life events such as pregnancy and birth. Positive expectations have proved important in our occupational health work, such as raising health and safety issues with those employees who have just been promoted. Drugs education in prisons (for example to avoid accidental overdoses) was best done in the two weeks before release from custody, when prisoners were able to contemplate the possibility of a happier life of freedom (Caan 1991).

For more than 20 years, researchers have been studying risk intensively and from many perspectives. The field of risk analysis has grown rapidly, focusing on issues of risk assessment and risk management. The former involves the identification, quantification and characterisation of threats to human health and the environment, while the latter, risk management, centres around processes of communication, mitigation and decision-making. But, as Slovic (1999) points out risk analysis is a political enterprise as well as a scientific one, in which public perception of risk also plays a role, bringing issues of values, process, power and trust into the picture. Risk perception may operate at both the level of individual behaviour and groups; for example, a group of penguins may dive off the ice together in the presence of a predator like a killer whale, when a single penguin will not go into the water. Groups sometimes initiate high risk behaviour, e.g. football hooligans, that as individuals they would be unlikely to chance.

Perceptions of risk play a prominent role in the decisions people make, in the sense that differences in risk perception lie at the heart of disagreements about the best course of action between technical experts and members of the general public (Slovic 1987), men and women (Flynn et al. 1994; Finucane et al. 2000; Weber et al. 2002) and people from different cultures (Weber and Hsee 1998; 1999). Both individual and group differences in preference for risky decision alternatives and situational differences in risk preference have been shown to be associated with differences in perceptions of the relative risk of choice options, rather than with differences in attitude towards (perceived) risk, that is, a tendency to approach or to avoid options perceived as riskier (Weber and Milliman 1997; Weber 2001a). Perceptions and misperceptions of risk, both by members of the public and by public officials, also appear to play a large role in the current examination of our preparedness to deal with health risks.

Risk issues can and do generate controversies. Readers need to keep an open mind about calculating the objective risks when only limited information is available. In many countries, severe conflicts about the evaluation of risks have emerged, particularly with respect to large-scale technologies such as nuclear energy and genetic engineering (Johnson and Covello 1987; von Winterfeldt and Edwards 1984; Beck 1992; Cvetkovich and Earle 1992). Uncertainly has generated considerable research on the topic of subjective risk perception. Our objective for this chapter is to examine the interplay between several individual factors, trends in society and globalisation pertaining to risk perception.

The authors have been asked for advice on health risks associated with the expansion of Stansted Airport on the outskirts of London. Objective information is in very short supply and debate tends to take emotionally charged and entrenched positions characterised by the 'drama triangle' of victim–persecutor–rescuer. These primitive roles can be adopted by children in family arguments but rarely lead to any resolution of the problem underlying the argument – rather they perpetuate the quarrel. One of the most powerful benefits in addressing communicating perceptions of risk is that people may cooperate to manage potential problems together. The alternative to addressing perceptions of risk is that people just end up have slanging matches, real problems are left unaddressed, and perceptions harden.

Risk perception

The term risk perception is generally taken to be the evaluation or judgement of the likelihood of harm. The severity of harm could range from mild and temporary injury, disease, to disintegration and death under specific circumstances. Objective evaluation usually involves concepts from probability such as odds, absolute and relative risks. However, this objective measure of risk does not tell the whole story and, in determining acceptability of any particular risk, perceived risk is likely to play a large role in people's judgements and evaluations of hazards which they (or their facilities, or the environment) are or might be exposed to.

For example, people's perceptions may be categorical – deadly, worth chancing and safe. Based on their interpretations of the world, experiences and beliefs, everybody is engaged with risk perception most of the time, whether driving a car or thinking about health care or deciding financial matters. Perceptions of a particular hazard are strongly influenced by how disastrous a negative consequence would be and how commonplace exposure to risk is. An asteroid destroying life on earth would be a catastrophe but is so outside people's everyday experience that it is very difficult for them to hold any objective judgement on it. However, this does not prevent some unfortunate individuals from developing a fear based on mass media around such a sensational event that it becomes a disability.

Childhood sexual abuse is quite a common phenomenon worldwide; for example six per cent of general practice patients can recall specific incidents of abuse. Perceptions of risk focus on abuse by strangers, usually outside the child's household ('paedophile pervs' in the headlines). While there is a finite risk of abuse outside the child's household the great majority of incidents recorded objectively involve familiar figures close to the child's home. The very commonplace nature of the risk of abusive relationships in the domestic setting makes it very difficult for someone like a grandparent to accept this possibility. By and large it is not the gym teacher who was recently subject of press frenzy (UK, January 2006).

Early studies of risk perception demonstrated that the public's concerns could not simply be blamed on ignorance or irrationality. Rather, research showed that many of the public's responses to risk could be attributed to uncertainty in risk assessments, perceived inequity in the distribution of risks and benefits and aversion to being exposed to risks that were involuntary, not under one's control or dreaded. In the 1980s, a group of researchers from Decision Research in Oregon led by Paul Slovic, Sarah Lichtenstein and Baruch Fischhoff, proposed a survey-based method for studying risk perception that remains influential today.

The importance of social values in risk perception and risk acceptance came to be recognised (Slovic 1987). The role of trust emerged as another important aspect of risk perception, management and significantly for this book, risk communication. To be effective, Slovic (2000) asserts that 'risk communicators must recognise and overcome a number of obstacles that have their roots in the limitations of scientific risk assessment and the idiosyncrasies of the human mind' (p.182). Risk perception by the public can be said to be built upon on a meta-judgement of risk based on multidimensional factors.

Understanding how people view risk is often as important as understanding the risk itself. Individuals sometimes have a very different perspective from experts. This is not always because of a different interpretation of the facts. In some cases, their views can be based on entirely different assumptions and values. Communication which sets out to change or influence beliefs without recognising the rational basis of those beliefs, or tries to divert attention away from people's real concerns, will almost certainly fail.

Culture heroes and risk perception

The term 'culture', discussed in Chapter 3, refers to 'the meanings that people learn from and share with each other' (MacPherson et al. 1989, 249). This includes descriptive and normative beliefs which are shared by members of the cultural group. 'Popular culture', therefore, can then be defined as the normative values and beliefs that are available for the general mass of people on a local, national or global scale. This culture has been referred to as 'low culture' as compared to 'high culture' which includes art, literature and opera (Lovat et al. 1994, 180).

The nature of popular culture changes over time as ideas of what is popular change within local, national or global communities. Such changes are driven by mass media such as television, film, music, magazines and the Internet. In fact, many of these media may be thought of as popular culture in themselves. These cultures generally are youthful and have shared values that are embodied by their own mythology, heroes, dress and jargon. Adverts, films and documentaries depict culture heroes such as surfers to be strong and determined heroic 'watermen' that risk their lives for the ultimate surfing experience.

The media industry makes the idea of 'living on the edge' into a consumer product. The extreme sports industry sells the image of aspiration: wear a 'Just do it' cap; drink a can of 'Live life to the max' Pepsi; talk on an X-Games mobile phone. This promotes the appearance of living on the edge, posing at taking risks while actually doing nothing at all. In the passive act of buying consumer goods, people are offered thrills and spills. It is not the real act of grappling with a challenge, but the image of 'pushing it to the MAX'. This is why extreme sports are so hyped up: the adrenaline factor is sold in concentrated form. But significantly, these images encourage some people to experiment with some extreme sports.

The sociological and anthropological literature documents that extreme sports are attracting an ever-increasing body of participants (see, for example Beal 1995; Humphreys 1997; Rinehart 1998a and 1998b; Palmer 1999 and 2002). Ranging from weekend warriors who do no training all year, have little skill and are content to infrequently subject themselves to the waves, the single tracks and the great outdoors, through to hard-core practitioners who are fully assimilated into their particular sport, fashion and technical skill of their preferred discipline, the extreme sports market, Palmer argues, is a hotchpotch of interests and expertise.

In response to this growing market of extreme sportspeople, a burgeoning media industry has inevitably flourished. Given the centrality of specialised equipment and associated paraphernalia to adventure sports, it is not surprising that a sizeable media industry now promotes a tantalising range of state-of-the-art sporting exotica. Gloves, sunglasses, helmets, T-shirts, sandshoes, protective padding, bikes, karabiners and surf wax are all on sale for the discerning extreme buyer. Even so-called 'alternative' youth cannot escape the pivotal commercial involvement in their sport. Beal, writing about social resistance in the subculture of skateboarding, notes that there are 'those involved in corporate bureaucratic skating as "rats"; individuals who brought the commercially produced paraphernalia and plastered all their belongings with corporate logos' (Beal 1995, 255). Thus, the landscape of contemporary sport is now smattered with the increasing presence of a range of commercial images and interests, and an examination of aspects of this media provides an ideal touchstone to some of the values and attitudes of those who engage in these frontier challenge activities.

At times various subcultures within popular culture may be seen as undesirable by the wider community because certain values and attitudes are emphasised such as drug use, as seen in the Ibiza phenomenon, or sexual promiscuity. However some subcultures of popular culture can influence mainstream culture, for example the environmental movement, and are in turn influenced by the mainstream, such as professionalism and commercialisation, as seen in the extreme sports arena. Taking the example of extreme sports, there is a paradoxical message – those who take the real risks and succeed are respected and applauded. These culture icons and culture heroes in turn trigger others, frequently amateurs, to engage in similar activities to gain some reflected glory. But many do not have the appropriate training or skills to engage on a tourist basis with the risks involved in such activities as white-water rafting or mountain climbing.

Meanwhile, large transnational corporations perpetuate popular cultures through the commodification and promotion of paraphernalia such as magazines, movies, computer games, accessories, equipment and clothing. Today, the selling of popular culture to the youth market fosters multi-billion-dollar industries on a global basis. These industries, using sophisticated technology, promote their products and paraphernalia to those who identify with that culture, exploiting the value and belief systems that culture has itself developed. In return that popular culture may grow from a small, localised counter culture, such as extreme sport, into a leisure pursuit or a way of life for thousands of people on a global basis.

Risk also includes the subjective evaluation of that risk, as seen in Table 4.1. A number of principles from the behavioural and social sciences guide how people make these evaluations. Risk perception determines the level of concern, worry, anger, fear, and hostility, which are the subjective factors that influence how people interpret a threat. How people respond emotionally to perceived hazards (Slovic et al. 1990) in turn affects their attitudes and subsequent behaviours.

Emotional intensity seems to influence significantly both risk-perception and risk-taking. On a comparatively low level of emotional intensity, emotions can be understood to be an

Table 4.1 Factors related to how we determine risk

Risk factor	Perceptions of risk will be greater when the threat is seen as:
Voluntariness	Involuntary or imposed
Controllability	Under the control of others
Familiarity	Unfamiliar
Equity	Unevenly and inequitably distributed
Benefits	Unclear or having questionable benefits
Understanding	Poorly understood
Uncertainty	Relatively unknown or having highly uncertain dimensions
Dread	Evoking fear, terror or anxiety
Reversibility	Having potentially irreversible adverse effects
Trust in institutions	Requiring credible institutional response
Personal stake	Placing people personally and directly at risk
Ethical/moral nature	Ethically objectionable or morally wrong
Human versus natural origin	Generated by human action (versus acts of God)
Victim identity	Producing victims that one can identify with
Catastrophic potential and temporarily	Producing fatalities/injuries/illness grouped spatially

Source: Slovic et al (1980)

'adviser' for decision making. The evaluation of one's feelings is then used to find out how to judge the risk (Loewenstein et al. 2001). In situations of a high level of emotions, cognitive consideration might be ruled out by emotions/affect. This reflects the observation that under specific circumstances, risk calculation as a whole is rejected (ibid.), for example, parents' response to the measles, mumps and rubella (MMR) vaccine. One of the reasons to refuse risk-taking is that probable outcomes are seen as so horrible or catastrophic that even the smallest probability is refused.

The main issues are whether a risk is acceptable to the public and if it is not acceptable, what is the scope for reducing risk. If a policy imposes a particular view about risks that people are not prepared to accept, then it is likely to be unpopular, difficult and costly to implement. If public concerns about a risk are not identified and aired early on, then these may escalate into a crisis. On the other hand, if people are indifferent to a risk because they feel that it does not affect them individually, then it may require considerable time and effort to motivate them to take action to tackle it.

Both risks and benefits have to be considered when seeking to understand what drives some behaviours and why some interventions are more acceptable and successful than others. Social, cultural and economic factors are central to how individuals perceive health risks. Similarly, societal and structural factors can influence which risk control policies are adopted and the impact that interventions can achieve. Preventing risk factors has to be planned within the context of local society, bearing in mind that the success of preventive interventions is only partly a matter of individual circumstances and education.

Perceptions of health risks in developing countries

Lifestyle risks to health, as an area for further study, have only recently begun to receive attention in developing countries according to the World Health Organization's World Health Report

2002. In a rich country like Britain many Government initiatives around health, for example 'Choosing Health' (Department of Health 2004), aim to reduce deaths before the pension age of 65 through lifestyle changes involving diet and exercise. In most developing countries, the life expectancy is well below 65 and in the World Bank least developed economies can be under 40. Therefore, perception of a healthy lifespan may be very different in communities where there is no expectation of reaching advanced age. The need to view health risks in their local context of daily threats, such as poverty, food insecurity and lack of income, is obvious when analysing perceptions of risk in these countries, particularly when lifestyle risk factors are considered alongside life-threatening diseases such as malaria, HIV/AIDS and the growing pandemic of tuberculosis. In addition, families may face many other important external risks, such as crushing poverty, political instability, wars, violence and of course natural disasters. Thus, for those living in the poorest countries of the world, there is a whole array of risks that have to be considered by individuals and families every day. Moreover, expectations and any sense of control to reduce risks may be different.

Lay understandings of risk are embedded in an evolving cultural process which resists categorisation within the static abstractions of 'grand theory' (Irwin et al. 1999, 1325). An example of how people interpret or understand risk is closely aligned to their experience of the world. In the following example one can clearly see that the experience of malaria in one part of Africa is such that the respondents take a global view of the causes and management of malaria.

In focus group discussions, women agreed that fever – referred to by the local terms such as koraye *and* abum *was a major health problem in the area. A variety of causes were identified, including the consumption of inappropriate food, failure to take enemas regularly, and as a result of working or sitting in the sun or other heat. A few agreed that mosquitoes caused fever, but only in response to a direct prompt: 'Mosquitoes eat dirty water and inject you with it' or 'Mosquitoes bite others with a disease and if they bite you later, can give you fever'.*

(Agyepong and Manderson 1999, 83)

Susan Cutter suggests that what becomes clear 'is not how much we know, but rather how little we know about how individuals and society perceive risk' (Cutter 1993, 23).

Models of individual risk perception and behaviour were, however, mainly developed in industrialised countries where people have considerably higher personal autonomy and freedom to act, better access to health information, and more scope for making choices for better health (WHO 2002). Some would argue that such models may be less appropriate in low and middle income countries, where illnesses and deaths are closely associated with poverty and infectious and communicable diseases (Manderson 2001). In industrialised countries, studies of HIV/AIDS and, to a lesser extent, non-communicable diseases such as cancer (Gifford, 1986) and coronary heart disease (Davison et al. 1991, 1–9) have been carried out using the perspectives of applied medical anthropology and sociology (Manderson and Tye 1997).

In developing countries where communicable diseases remain the main cause of avoidable mortality, these disciplines have most frequently been used to help evaluate the effectiveness of disease control programmes. Perceptions of disease, use of health services and reasons for non-compliance are some areas often studied (Pelto and Pelto 1997).

For communicable diseases, it is important to differentiate perceptions of the risk of a disease from those concerned with the risk of acquiring the infection, particularly as not all infections, such as sexually transmitted infections and tuberculosis, will develop into symptomatic disease. Interrupting transmission of infections, for example through the use of measles vaccine or bed nets in malaria control, is the main way in which control programmes reduce risk. In such situations, risks are often determined from the point of view of whether an effective response exists in practice. Thus, effectiveness evaluation is based on such indicators as early recognition of signs for severe illness (for example, acute respiratory infections), symptoms requiring self-referral for treatment (for example, leprosy and schistosomiasis), or use of impregnated bed nets to prevent malaria transmission. Much of this anthropological research for effectiveness evaluation has been supported by multilateral agencies and bilateral donors, including WHO and UNAIDS.

Because of the effects of the demographic and epidemiological transitions, many middle- and low-income developing country populations face existing risks from communicable diseases, as well as rapid increases in risks to health from many risk factors and non-communicable diseases. Although avoidance of risks of infection, often perceived as risk of disease, are implicit in most biomedical and public health models of disease control in developing countries, more research from the anthropological point of view is clearly needed to place these risks in perspective among a whole array of other risks to life. Given competing risks, it cannot be assumed that if people are better informed on their exposures to risk factors they will necessarily act to change their health behaviours.

Influences on risk perceptions and decision-making

Two important factors that influence risk perception are gender and world views, with affiliation, emotional affect and trust also being strongly correlated with the risk judgements of experts as well as lay persons. The influence of gender has been well documented, with men tending to judge risks as smaller and less problematic than do women. Explanations have focused mainly on biological and social factors. For example, it has been suggested that women are more socialised to care for human health and are less likely to be familiar with science and technology. However, female toxicologists were found to judge the same risks as higher than do male toxicologists (Barke et al. 1997; Slovic et al. 1997). In another study dealing with perception of 25 hazards, males produced risk-perception ratings that were consistently much lower than those of females (Flynn et al. 1994). To the extent that socio-political factors shape public perception of risks, gender differences appear to have an important effect on interpreting risks.

The influence of social, psychological and political factors can also be seen in studies on the impact of world views on risk judgements. World views are general social, cultural and political attitudes that appear to have an influence over people's judgements about complex issues (Dake 1991). World views include feelings such as fatalism towards control over risks to health, belief in hierarchy and leaving decisions to the experts, and a conviction that individualism is an important characteristic of a fair society, or that technological developments are important for improving our health and social well-being. These world views have been found to be strongly linked to public perceptions of risk (Peters and Slovic 1996). These views have also been the subject of a few international studies, for example comparing perceptions of risks to nuclear power in the United States with those in other industrialised countries (Jasper 1990).

Risk decision-making

In many situations people are required to deal with more details than they can readily handle at any one time. To avoid overload, people tend to simplify. They want to know whether foods are safe, rather than treating safety as a continuous variable; they demand proof from scientists who can only provide tentative conclusions concerning safety; and they divide the participants in risk disputes into good guys and bad guys. Such simplifications help people to cope with risk decision-making but can also lead to biases (Kahneman et al. 1982).

Once people's minds are made up, it is often difficult to change them unless confronted with overwhelming evidence to the contrary. One psychological process that helps people to maintain their current beliefs is underestimating the need to seek contrary evidence. Another process is exploiting the uncertainty surrounding negative information to interpret it as consistent with existing beliefs (Gilovich 1993).

Moreover, people are good at keeping track of events that come to their attention (Peterson and Beach 1967; Hasher and Zacks 1984, 356–88). Consequently, if appropriate facts reach people from a credible source and in a credible way before their minds are made up, their first impression is more likely to be the correct one. It is difficult, however, for people to acquire first-hand knowledge of many risks, leaving them to decipher whatever incomplete information they may have access to.

Importantly, people cannot readily detect omissions in the evidence they receive, nor recognise that their own observations may be biased. Thus people's risk perceptions can be manipulated in the short term by selective presentations. People will not know and may not sense how much has been left out (Fischhoff et al. 1978). What happens in the long term depends on whether the missing information is revealed by other experiences or sources.

For some risk experts, the natural unit of risk is an increase in probability of death; for others, it is a reduced life expectancy; for still others, it is the scale of deaths in relation to exposure. Since lay people and risk managers tend to use the term risk differently, they may agree on the facts of a hazard or risk, but disagree about its riskiness (Slovic et al. 1979, 14–20, 36–9; Fischhoff et al. 1984, 123–39; Fischhoff and Svenson 1988, 453–71). Risk decision-making is often taken within the context of local beliefs and values. The following case study illustrates this point.

Local beliefs: the case of malaria

Malaria is a major public health problem in Malawi, under-five children and pregnant women being the most vulnerable. Munthali's (2005) study, undertaken among the Tumbuka of northern Malawi, details the perceptions about the aetiology, treatment and prevention of malaria in under-five children. One of the major findings is that while Fansidar is currently the treatment for malaria, there are delays in seeking the right treatment because of, among other factors, perceptions about the cause of malaria: therefore children were only taken to the health centre when traditional medicines failed.

Munthali (2005) reported that while most young women recognised that malaria is caused by mosquitoes, they also said that there are other causes of malaria, for example the exposure of the child to very cold weather (*kuzizima chomene*) and the consumption of very cold foods. Informants said that the consumption of cold foods and exposure of the child to very cold weather make the child feel cold and start shivering, consequently they will develop fever.

Shivering and fever are perceived to be symptoms of malaria (according to informants) and this is why they conclude that cold weather and eating very cold foods can also cause malaria.

Based on this explanatory model, one would expect that there should be a very high incidence and prevalence of malaria in June and July when Malawi has a winter season, however, most mothers in this study reported that while there are a lot of children suffering from malaria during winter, most of the cases of malaria occur in the rainy season, but they failed to link the high prevalence of malaria with the high population of mosquitoes in the rainy season.

People have their own perceptions about malaria and its accompanying signs and symptoms, which shape their decisions on prevention and therapy seeking (see Brain 1990; Agyepong 1992; Foster 1995; Baume et al. 2000). For example, Brain claims that during the 1929–1933 malaria epidemics in Natal and Zululand, people were influenced by the traditional healers to refuse to take quinine, claiming that the government wanted to kill them, that quinine would cause impotence and sterility, and that in fact quinine caused malaria (Brain 1990). The risks from the disease were considered much less than the risks of poisoning by the government or impotency. The bitterness of chloroquine and its subsequent association with the bitter traditional abortifacients created a negative correlation in the minds of people that outweighed the purportive benefits of the drug.

The lack of money to purchase anti-malarial drugs (see Foster 1995) set up dilemmas for those already seriously impoverished about what to spend what little money they have on. Moreover, the claim that Fansidar worsens the condition of patients suffering from malaria (Matinga and Munthali 2001) are some of the factors that influences risk perception and decision-making in developing countries. Many people, both in the developed and developing world take a fatalistic attitude towards the prevention of disease (Munthali 2005, 7).

Understanding people's perceptions of malaria, and the factors which influence these perceptions, must be a central part of mounting successful interventions to control malaria throughout the world (Bradley et al. 1991; Lipowsky, et al, 1992; Ahorlu et al. 1997). People in different societies hold a variety of beliefs about the cause and transmission of malaria that vary according to cultural, educational, and economic factors, and have direct consequences for both preventive and treatment-seeking behaviour as well as for activities to control malaria. But this conundrum cannot be viewed simplistically, since a solution to misguided perceptions, in terms of current public health knowledge, is not just a matter of providing correct knowledge. As Espino et al. have noted, 'Improving or increasing knowledge does not necessarily result in changes in perceptions or behaviour' (Espino et al. 1997, 237). Indeed, behaviour is not just a consequence of knowledge and belief: levels of alcoholism, community, social and political divisions, or lack of control by women of household budgets, for example, are also significant determinants (Agyepong and Manderson 1999, 79).

Overview

Based on research, specific factors that influence public risk perception include:

- control   the ability of the individual or society to control the risk;
- catastrophic potential – the possibility of fatalities or ill effects grouped in time and space as in an epidemic;
- dread – the fear of the possibility of serious delayed effects, such as cancer;

- familiarity – the degree of familiarity lay people have with the risk;
- equity – refers to the equal distribution of risks and benefits throughout society;
- level of knowledge – the general understanding lay people have with the process or activity posing the risk;
- voluntariness of exposure;
- effects on children and future generations – concerns about possible delayed effects on humans and the environment posed by the risk;
- clarity of benefits – represents the awareness and understanding of the benefits provided by the activity posing the risk;
- media attention;
- trust in organisations or institutions.

The public uses these characteristics to judge the acceptability of a risk rather than using risk estimates based on experiments. For example, the public views genetically modified (GM) crops that produce food as riskier to their health than the natural carcinogens in common foods and beverages because they believe they have no control over their exposure to the GM foods they are consuming. Additionally, people may tolerate the risks from chemicals inherent in food, but they are unwilling to tolerate additional risks from biotechnology ingredients, no matter how small. People tend to accept the risks from driving an automobile much more readily than the risks from GM foods because they have control over the automobile.

How people view risks and apply value judgements is perhaps the most challenging factor to take into account when developing an approach to the health risk communication, not least because these views and value judgements are not static but change according to circumstances. We have evolved to cope with the dangers and uncertainty of life; we have in-built mechanisms for dealing with risk – mechanisms that reflect our personal preferences and the values of the society in which we live.

Conclusion

The purpose of risk communication by professionals is to enable people to avoid harm. The success of communicating a particular risk to a lay audience depends on shifting their perceptions which involves a complex interaction between the characteristics of the audience, the source of the message and its content. As well as the dialogue between professional and lay participants, communication is often shaped by properties of the hazard itself, particularly dimensions of controllability, familiarity and an attribution to natural events or to human hubris.

5 The Art and Science of Health Risk Communication
by Dawn Hillier

In this chapter we turn our attention to contrasting styles and approaches to health risk communication: the literary didactic approach, appealing to logic; the interactive media that fosters audience participation in television and radio programmes; and online self-assessment of personal risk (health) products are contrasted with, for example, risk communication styles that adopt the storytelling approach using drama, dialogue and acting to generate active participation of audience, drawing on examples from fieldwork in Africa.

There is a great deal written about communicating risk to the public that draws on more than three decades of research. There is no intention in this chapter to present a comprehensive review of risk communication. Rather, I shall focus on a number of what seems to me to be the salient issues: public involvement in risk communication; liminal and subliminal risk messages in popular cultural artefacts, such as soap operas and chat shows; risk images, the role of the media, storytelling and professional risk communication.

For the purposes of this chapter we decided to adopt the definition of risk communication suggested by Covello et al. (1986): risk communication is defined as any purposeful exchange of information about health or environment risks between interested parties. More specifically, risk communication is the act of conveying or transmitting information to interested parties about (a) levels of health or environmental risks; (b) the significance or meaning of health or environmental risks; or (c) decisions, actions or policies aimed at managing or controlling health or environmental risks. Interested parties, according to Covello et al. (1986, 172), include government agencies, industry and corporations, trade unions, the media, scientists, professional organisations, public interest groups and individual citizens.

Risk management has become a dominant concern of public policy and yet the ability of government to anticipate the strength and focus of public concerns remains weak. Rectifying the misunderstandings and assuaging the deep anxieties that surround health risk scares can, and does, cost governments billions of pounds (Breakwell and Barnett 2001). It is vital, therefore to understand the genesis and development of such risk impacts in order to generate trust and credibility. These are central to effective communication about topics of high concern. Consequently, this chapter focuses on theories and practices of health risk communication, particularly drawing out differing approaches used to communicate risks in facts as given by the scientific, governmental and non-governmental agencies, stories, allegories, rumours, metaphors and images, and personal examples (the concern here is to explore how humans communicate naturally); and to explore how health risk is communicated in popular cultural artefacts, such as the media, in different countries and cultural groups.

The art and science of professional risk communication

Professional risk communication is a science-based approach for communicating effectively in high-concern situations – it provides a set of principles and tools for meeting those challenges. It evolved from psychometric risk perception studies, associated most notably with the American researcher Paul Slovic and his co-workers. At first, risk communication research was seen as a government tool to develop information programmes to increase the public's knowledge of environmental health and technological hazards to which they were exposed. This was referred to as top-down risk communication. After researchers pointed out that experts too are fallible and biased, the field moved toward reciprocal risk communication to promote dialogue between the public and experts to derive solutions acceptable to everyone.

Effective communication is critical to the successful resolution of any type of health, safety, or environmental controversy (Slovic 1987; Covello et al. 1989; National Research Council 1989). High-concern situations involving risk create substantial barriers to effective communication (Fischhoff 1995; Covello 1998) and evoke strong emotions, such as fear, anxiety, distrust, anger, outrage, helplessness and frustration (Sandman 1989; Covello and Sandman 2001). When the communication environment becomes emotionally charged, the rules for effective communication change. Familiar and traditional approaches often fall short or can make the situation worse (Covello, et al 1989; National Research Council 1989).

Effective health risk communication is a combination of art and science. Science usually defines risk in relation to large populations, but people seldom see such probabilities as applying directly to themselves. The art is enabling individuals to see the risks as they apply to themselves. In order for this to happen, professional health risk communication is seen as transdisciplinary in nature, drawing upon multiple disciplines (World Health Organization 2003; Bernhardt 2004). Professional health communicators recognise the complexity of attaining behaviour and social change and use a multi-faceted approach that is grounded in the application of several theoretical frameworks (highlighted in Chapter 4) and disciplines, including but not being limited to health education, social marketing, and behavioural and social change theories. Effective health risk communication draws upon principles that have been successfully used in the private and commercial sectors but also upon the audience-centred approach of other disciplines, such as psychology, sociology, anthropology (World Health Organization 2003), and cultural and media studies. It is less anchored to a single specific theory or model.

Piotrow et al. (2003, 1–2) identified four different 'eras' of health communication:

1 the clinic era, based on a medical care model and the notion that if people knew where services were located they would find their way to their clinics;
2 the field era, a more proactive approach emphasising outreach workers, community-based distribution, and a variety of information, education, and communication (IEC) products;
3 the social marketing era, developed from the commercial concepts that consumers will buy the products they want at subsidised prices;
4 the era of strategic behaviour communications, founded on behavioural science models that emphasise the need to influence social norms and policy environments as to facilitate and empower the iterative and dynamic process of both individual and social change.

Even in the context of strategic behaviour communications, however, many of the theoretical approaches of the different eras of health communication may well be used in programme planning or execution. Keeping the audience at the centre of each intervention in health risk communication is essential, applying a case-by-case approach in selecting those models, theories and strategies that are best suited to:

- reach people's hearts and minds;
- secure their involvement in the health issue and its solutions;
- support and facilitate the journey to reduce or contain the risk.

While health educators tend to focus primarily on changing health beliefs (Andreasen 1995), professional health communicators consider that educating target audiences about health issues is only the first step of a long-term audience-centred process. This process often requires theoretical flexibility to accommodate the needs of differing audiences. Health risk communication demands that communicators focus not only on channels, messages and tools but attempt to persuade, involve and create consensus and feelings of ownership among interested parties.

As in social marketing, those concerned should be involved in planning, testing and implementing key strategies, messages and activities. However, the planning framework for this process does not solely rely on marketing techniques and theories, it also applies more traditional communication models, such as the communication for persuasion theory (McGuire 1984) and several other social science, mass communication and health education theories (Institute of Medicine 2003; Health Communication Partnership 2005; World Health Organization 2003).

In designing intervention strategies, it cannot automatically be assumed that the diverse groups which make up the general public think in the same way as public health professionals and other risk experts. In addition, estimates of risk and its consequences, presented in scientific terms based on a risk assessment, have to be communicated with particular caution and care. The World Health Organization (2002) considers that the best way is for well-respected professionals, who are seen to be independent and credible, to make the communications. An atmosphere of trust between the government and all interested parties, in both the public and private sectors, is essential if interventions are to be adopted and successfully implemented.

Undertaking adequate risk communication means finding ways of presenting information that is complex and sometimes technical, often clouded by uncertainty and inherently difficult to understand. For example, let us consider the following case.

Case example: risk communication – New York City's West Nile virus response

The first outbreak of West Nile virus[1] in New York City occurred in late summer 1999. When the virus broke out, callers flooded public health phone lines asking questions such as whether

---

1   Most cases are mild, with people showing no symptoms or having a fever, headache and body aches. Other symptoms include a mild rash, swollen lymph glands, severe headache, high fever, stiff neck, confusion, seizures, aversion to light, muscle weakness and loss of consciousness. It is thought that infected people develop a lifelong immunity to the disease. In the New York outbreak, 67 people became ill. By 14 August 1999, 156 human cases of West Nile virus encephalitis or meningitis had been reported and nine people had died, according to the US Centers for Disease Control and Prevention (CDC). Only 14 cases were reported in 2000 and 2001.

children should play outdoor soccer. Those bitten by mosquitoes were rushed to emergency departments and schools cancelled outdoor field trips.

Anxiety was high when the disease made its first appearance in the Western Hemisphere. A state-wide West Nile virus risk communications workgroup was established and by the following summer, the New York City Department of Health had developed a detailed response plan that included public education and outreach (New York City Department of Health 2000). The three objectives for public education and outreach plan were:

1   to improve the public's awareness of risk for disease;
2   to improve the public's participation in eliminating potential breeding sites; and
3   to provide timely and accurate information related to insecticide spraying.

Covello et al (2001) reported that channels of communication included television and radio public service announcements; press releases, extensive media outreach, and announcements during the scheduled daily Mayoral press conferences; brochures and fact sheets, prepared in 10 to 15 languages; posters placed throughout the city; bill inserts mailed with the cooperation of city utilities; 24-hour phone lines at the height of the outbreak, including the handling of over 150000 calls; a website that included general information, a question-and-answer section, forms for reporting standing water and dead birds, insecticide fact sheets, and press releases issued during the outbreak; and a number of town hall public meetings.

The primary spokespersons were the New York City Health Commissioner and the Mayor (or the Borough President in the outer boroughs). The majority of the press releases concerned spraying and included contact details numbers for further information. Print materials, generally written at a high school reading level, contained information about personal protective behaviour (for example, protection against mosquitoes). The public were also requested to assist government agencies by eliminating sources of standing water where mosquitoes might breed.

Covello et al. (2001) consider that in general, the New York City risk communication effort related to the West Nile virus epidemic was far-reaching, resource intensive, competently handled and effective. However, they note that improvements can be made in several areas. For example, New York City officials were clearly aware of risk perception factors and took these factors into account in their decisions. Conversely, apparently little effort was made to collect, analyse and evaluate empirical information (obtained through focus groups and surveys) about stakeholder judgements of each of the major risk perception factors.

Furthermore, the full range of communication channels, such as information exchanges and information workshops, for engaging stakeholders in sustained interaction about identified areas of concern were not exploited. Official spokespersons were apparently not informed about stakeholder perceptions or about various stakeholder groups' expected levels of concern, fear, hostility or outrage. Public concern over the City's decision to use pesticides for vector control, as well as the controversial decision to engage in aerial spraying by highly visible helicopters, underscores what appears to be an initial failure by City officials to ascertain the risk perceptions of an expanded circle of stakeholders, including wildlife experts and environmental groups (Covello et al. 2001).

In their analysis, Covello and colleagues determined that the communication materials produced by City officials were highly informative. However, from a mental noise perspective, they:

- contained many more messages than could be easily comprehended by the intended audience;
- contained inadequate repetition and visualisation. For example, explanatory charts and graphs were generally absent, as were video tapes about the effects of the West Nile virus;
- were several school grade-levels higher than recommended.

Covello et al.'s (2001) analysis of West Nile virus case study material indicates an apparent lack of attention to the unequal weights given to negative and positive information in high-concern situations. For example, many of the communications focused more on what was not being done by City authorities, than on what was being done. In addition, negative messages (for example, the decision to spray pesticides from helicopters and the decision to cancel a concert at Central Park) were not counterbalanced by a larger number of positive or solution-oriented messages. Moreover, there was little evidence that the positive or solution-oriented messages that were offered were the product of sustained interaction and dialogue with a wide range of stakeholders.

Additional factors compounded trust problems. The telephone hotlines, for example, while answered 24 hours a day, were, in some cases, staffed by personnel who were inadequately trained in risk communication. Communication directed to sensitive populations, such as people with asthma, about spraying locations and schedules was neglected. Additionally, town hall meetings were over-utilised, while more effective small group activities, such as information exchanges and public workshops, were under-utilised.

Emerging diseases, such as SARS and Asian Flu, along with risks of bioterrorism present extraordinary risk communication challenges. Consequently, it is important to develop an effective risk communication strategy for such eventualities. It would be a serious error as Covello et al. remind us, to underestimate the importance of engaging in dialogue among stakeholders and developing by consensus the final communication strategy and plan.

Risk images and risk communication

Unlike formal analytical risk assessments that may underpin the risk communicator's conclusions about a risk, the typical member of the public makes risk-related decisions without the help of written records, calculations, systematic reviews of scientific literature and other tools to aid decision-making. How people make decisions about risks such as evaluating whether something is a personal threat and deciding what actions should be taken is more often than not based on experience and memory. The operation of working memory controls what new information a person will attend to, access to information in long-term memory, and the mental operations performed on both. A key process in the operation of working memory is the use of images (Cvetkovich and Earle 1991, 329).

Risk images offer us representations of knowledge about a hazard, reflections of an individual's mental models of a hazard which are used for making hazard evaluations. Image generation is a multi-process operation (see Kosslyn 1988) comprising framing, retrieval and image generation, inference, images, judgement and behaviour. A specific example may serve to illustrate the process. Consider, for example, how one might answer the following question, 'What would happen if Canvey Island[2] was flooded again?' Following a computer analogy of

---

2   Canvey Island in South East England – in the early hours of the morning on 1 February 1953, millions of tons of salt water broke through the dykes protecting low-lying Canvey from the sea and foamed

the basic operations of information processing (cf., Wyer and Srull 1986), Cvetkovich and Earle (1991) suggest that arriving at an answer follows a pattern of framing, retrieval and image generation, and inference.

In framing, the first step in considering a question of risk is the identification of the question's frame or the problem. Working memory identifies an answer to the question 'What is the problem?' The public do not always frame a problem in the same way as the risk communicator (Cvetkovich et al. 1987). Depending on the identified frame, possible answers to a question about flooding on Canvey Island might include descriptions of changes to the sea level, security of the flood barriers, effects on individuals, homes, furniture and furnishings, pets, costs of repairs, effects on farming and cattle, businesses and economic effects and descriptions of the possible course of action, such as methods of escape or some combination of these and other possibilities.

In retrieval and image generation, according to Cvetkovich and Earle (1991), a search of long-term memory takes place for appropriate mental models. A mental model contains information identifying conceptual variables and their relationship to each other. This knowledge may be either general in nature (Will we have sufficient warning?) or it may be specific to the problem in hand (Have I time to take up the carpets?[3]). An image of 'What would happen if Canvey flooded again?' is generated based on the information and structure of the activated mental model. In some cases the image represents the complete mental model while in other cases the size of the model and the limits of the size of working memory allow only part of the model to be activated at one time.

Conclusions are based on the image. For example, some people model flooding as risk to life and others as risk to property or livelihood. These two models might be expected to lead to somewhat different descriptions of the sequence of increases in flood waters following the breakdown of the flood barriers on Canvey Island. A mental image can also be used for making inferences to arrive at 'single point' evaluations such as risk estimations and for decision making (for example, Should I move off the Island now?).

As cited in Cvetkovich and Earle (1991, 331–332) extensive evidence has been collected demonstrating that visual images serve to store short-term memories which can be examined to answer informational questions and to make decisions. This becomes very important in the context of health risk communication since thinking and image processing have dramatic effects on risk judgments and future likelihood estimations, imagining that events will happen (Carroll 1978; Gregory et al. 1982) and giving explanations for hypothetical events. Anderson (1983) has also shown that the effects of imagining behavioural scripts can either increase or decrease intentions to perform a behaviour depending upon whether the imagined script has the actor performing or not performing it. Image rehearsal probably affects behaviour because it has the power to clarify and increase memory ability of the actions that could be taken in reaching the target behaviour (Gregory et al. 1982).

---

through streets of sleeping residents. Fifty-eight people died – the worst single British casualty figure in a tragedy which killed 1932 people along the English and Dutch North Sea coasts. Canvey is now effectively a fortress, protected against the sea by a ring of steel and concrete so formidable that its population has increased from just over 11000 before the flood to about 37000 now. All Canvey homes are built on a concrete raft.

3   Mrs Moffat's account of the flood – Mother tried to save carpets. 'I remember the night well, awoken by Councillor Mason who was shouting, "The island has been flooded." We all got up and my mother took up carpets where she could. Being in the hours of darkness, we were unable to realise the extent of the damage and what was happening, until daylight. The next day, we saw the damage with water all around us and we were told we must leave the island.' www.thisisessex.co.uk/essex/canveyfloods/mrsmoffatt. html.

The image–judgement–action information processing model implies respect for the functionality of citizens' responses claims Cvetkovich and Earle (1991, 340). The model also suggests that risk communicators should not assume that they can accurately predict public reactions. It would seem appropriate in many situations that the first step in risk communication should, therefore, be to discover how an audience (and its sub-groups) frame the risk problem and process, via mental models, information about the health risk. One of the key issues is that risk communicators often frame the risk more narrowly than do their audiences, assuming that the characteristics of health risks are defined solely by their physical characteristics or health consequences. People tend to make judgements about health risks that extend beyond the physical characteristics to include social processes related to the identification, control and mitigation of risks. Credibility and trust have a social, historical and political dimension, as well as a dimension of technical expertise. Framing a risk should therefore include physical risks, its social amplification and community processes.

Risk communication and the media

In many cases the media will be the main channel of communication with the wider public. It will be one of the biggest influences on how they perceive risk; and it is likely to have the greatest impact on them.

Media can play a significant role: raising awareness of the issues within government and civil society, engaging civil society in debate, interrogating policy and debating alternatives, promoting transparency in policy making and implementation, and building political commitment to include communication policies. However, at present the media do not generally have the capacity to play this role. Few journalists and editors are familiar enough with the issues to report and analyse them effectively, and communication is not seen as a priority for coverage.

Moreover, the media does not comprise a single organisation or have a single purpose. It has different purposes, different audiences and different concerns. Generally speaking the media comprises of national daily and Sunday newspapers, regional and local dailies, Sundays and weeklies, national and regional television, national and local radio, national and local media for ethnic communities, news agencies (such as Reuters, Press Association) and the international media – general and specialist publications produced at weekly, monthly and quarterly frequencies. The broadcast media is made up of 24-hour news programmes, national news bulletins, regional and local news bulletins, drive-time programmes, phone-ins, audience participation programmes (such as *Question Time*) and chat shows. Within these are editors, news editors, leader writers, columnists, correspondents who specialise in specific subjects (health, science, home affairs, industry and politics), general reporters, documentary writers and producers.

In a study undertaken by Breakwell and Barnett (2001) the media interviews revealed a series of factors that influence how a story involving risk is covered and shape the decision-making processes involved. These included: commercial pressures on the media to promote scare stories; they seek to provide 'infotainment'; consequently they avoid reporting 'real science'; the culture allows individual journalists and editors to pursue private agendas in reporting hazards; codes of practice in the media accentuate amplification processes; the absence of investigative journalism fuels a desire for information which is accessible and predigested; different arms of the media have different priorities; pressures groups work the media well; and the media like controversy and uncertainty – they are audience-grabbers.

The media tend to be the gatekeepers for ideas and the conduit for scares. Despite the growing diversity of information sources, for example the Internet, it is still true that the power to decide what the public should know rests with a fairly small number of newspaper publishers, editors and television and radio producers. For complex issues that involve multidisciplinary scientific input, this power is even more concentrated in one person (for example a health editor), who might determine the particular viewpoint of an entire magazine or television channel. Gatekeepers not only decide what detail we receive, but through their own language and imagery, they influence what we are likely to remember of these complex issues.

These gatekeepers have changed over time. In the mid 1950s writers and broadcasters, in many respects, were simply retailers of science, presenting prepared packages of information to readers and listeners. As readers became more sophisticated and the outlook of the times changed, journalists began to let personal opinion colour their interpretation of the science. By the 1960s journalists were discussing the mixed blessings of science and by the mid 1970s the environmental and consumer movements prompted speculation on the potential risks to human health from new technology. This speculation was further fuelled by several technological disasters: the Bhopal and Seveso chemical spills, the explosion of the space shuttle Challenger and the nuclear explosion at Chernobyl.

Since then there has been a divergence of public opinion on new technology. Generally, the public views a new medical technology as a good thing – a breakthrough – and is happy to discount drawbacks and reasonably discuss any moral and ethical issues surrounding it. But most other new technologies are scrutinised and criticised for even the smallest environmental or public health threat, the usual public reaction being fear and resistance to the change.

Gigli (2004) explains that proliferation and globalisation of the media have meant that young people in many countries now have increased – and increasing – access to various multi-media options, such as computer and video games, radio, printed material, and satellite and terrestrial TV channels. Specifically, Gigli claims that:

- Television is the dominant medium for young people worldwide. She provides figures from 21 countries indicating that from the mid 1980s to the mid 1990s, the number of TV channels, household TV sets and hours spent watching TV had more than doubled. Average daily use of this medium among those school-age children around the world with access ranges from between 1.5 hours to more than four hours.

- Radio is the next most popular medium among this age group, despite the fact that actual listening rates vary greatly between countries. In many places (for example Africa and the former Soviet Union), there has been a spike in the number of youth listeners. Gigli emphasises young people's interest in political and social events, and articulates the need for high-quality information.

- The Internet is also increasingly popular as a source of information, entertainment and communication among young people, especially among young men in the developed world.

- Print media is not experiencing the steady rise seen among young users of these other media. Gigli speculates that improvement in the quality and quantity of information available in other formats (in industrialised countries) or limited circulation and/or expense (in poorer countries) are among the factors responsible for this decline or levelling. Publications that appeal to young people's special interests, such as magazines focused on computers or music, tend to have the strongest pull.

Chapter 9 contains examples of how soap operas and chat shows have been used to communicate risk.

Conclusion

We are reminded daily that we are experiencing an 'information revolution', that since the second half of the twentieth century we have been living in an 'information society' and that in the twenty-first century we have to find our place in a 'knowledge society'. This shift in the social functions of information focuses on the dialectic between a growing demand for specific knowledge and the development of powerful and dynamic technologies for generating, storing and communicating information. Individual understanding of information and knowledge as commodities, tools or social goods whose transmission is central to social production and reproduction, and the associated concepts of information networks, systems and regimes, however, is dependent on location, experience and expertise (as far as the ability to access, and the freedom to use not only the technology but also the knowledge). The underlying questions of who gets to know what, and how, and how this affects the way life is lived, remain pressing ones for professional as well as lay risk communicators.

The impact of risk communication depends upon a complex interaction between the characteristics of the audience, the source of the message, and its content. Audience perception of risk is influenced by demographic factors (for example age and gender), personality profile, past experience and ideological orientation. It is also affected by cognitive biases (for example unrealistic optimism) and lay 'mental models' of the hazard. For food hazards, the important dimensions of risk are controllability, novelty and naturalness. The source must be trusted for a risk message to be effective. Trust is associated with believing the source is expert, unbiased, disinterested and not sensationalising. To maximise impact, risk communications must have a content which triggers attention, achieves comprehension and can influence decision making. It must be unambiguous, definitive and easily interpretable – rarely achievable particularly when risk is shrouded in scientific uncertainty. Risk messages initiate social processes of amplification and attenuation; consequently their ramifications are rarely controllable.

Today's obsession with risk management focuses too intently on the instruments of the management and measurement of risk. The more we delve into the jumble of equations and models the more we lose sight of the mystery of life. All too often, reason cannot answer. Even the most brilliant of mathematical geniuses will never be able to tell us what the future holds. In the end, what matters is the quality of our decisions in the face of uncertainty.

In communicating the risk and the risk reduction options in an effective, credible and timely manner, there is a need to consider:

- extreme complexity of risk factors;
- complexity of modeling and levels of uncertainty;
- complexity of lag effects and inertia;
- complexity of assessing roles and responsibilities of all global actors in relation to individual countries;

- problems in understanding cost estimates from economic modeling.

The key elements in effective risk communication are trust and credibility, caring and empathy, honesty and openness, competence and expertise and ultimately commitment and dedication. Therefore, the process of communicating health risks to the public must alternate listening and doing – research and action. The communicator enters into a dialogue with the community through the use of ongoing systematic research with representatives of the target audience.

6 Amplification of Risk: Styles and Approaches to Contemporary Health Risk Communication
by Mary Northrop, Dawn Hillier and Poonam Thapa

Drawing on examples from different countries, we will explore different approaches used in risk communication through contemporary hot topics such as, communicable diseases, sexual health, and obesity that serve to amplify and attenuate the risks involved. The chapter has been written in three 'voices': Mary Northrop explores the issues surrounding obesity to exemplify risk amplification and attenuation; Dawn Hillier delves into communicable diseases from a cultural-political perspective; and Poonam Thapa provides an analysis of sexual risk and proposes a different landscape for safe sex.

'If I'm going to sin then I might as well have cream on it!'

As I was standing behind a woman in a sandwich shop I overheard her saying to the woman serving her – 'I'll have a bacon sandwich please – and if I am going to sin, I might as well have white bread.' What has the world come to when a middle-aged woman sees the consumption of simple, nutritious food that has been eaten for centuries, as a flirtation with depravity? She may have been jesting but behind the remark lay a real fear that has been distilled by the endless pronouncements of food gurus and the medical profession. The diet industry is one of the most extraordinary phenomena of our times. Obesity has been elevated to the status as one of the deadly sins. One possible reason for this is that the medical profession has a tendency to medicalise behaviour we do not approve of (also seen in sexual health debates). As a result huge numbers of diet books are published every year. In just one morning watching television, there were four programmes broadcast concerning obesity demonstrating the current media frenzy around body weight.

Every day, new health studies fill the media, many of them often contradicting each other and earlier research. For years, women were told that hormone replacement therapy could reduce their risk of heart disease, stroke and Alzheimer's; now, new research finds that it may actually increase the risk for these disorders. Fish is a wonderful source of protein and Omega-3 fatty acids, which may reduce the risk of heart disease. But other studies claim that many fish are contaminated with high levels of mercury. Chocolate: artery-clogging bad guy or artery-clearing hero?

Over the last few years there has been growing concern over both the production and consumption of food: concerns over genetically modified crops came to prominence in the 1990s; the use of pesticides and the loss of nutritional values from foods have also been highlighted. Fears regarding the risk of contamination of food products such as salmonella from eggs, BSE from cows and mercury in fish have all contributed to questioning of the food we eat.

Today, this is added to by greater awareness of both nutrients and additional products within the food we consume. Nutrients may be added to food or water supplies but also removed from products via the production process. Additional products may be deliberately, accidentally or unknowingly added, either through production or the way in which food is prepared. The identification of 'good' and 'bad' fats, E numbers, the use of additives and food allergies are all relevant examples.

How do these issues come to be communicated and acknowledged as risks by individuals, governments and global communities?

Kasperson et al. (2001) present a framework for analysing stigma and social amplification of risk. Hazards become amplified for two reasons: they may be a new hazard not previously identified or an existing hazard that is more severe or difficult to manage than expected. One aspect of these socially amplified hazards is that they have the potential to generate stigma-related effects for places, technologies or products. This stigma then creates adverse effects thus multiplying the initial consequences. Kasperson et al. define the current usage of stigma as referring to 'an attribute of people, places, technologies or products that is deeply discrediting or devaluing. Instead of the possessor being viewed as normal or commonplace, the possessor is viewed as different, with this difference involving important qualities that set the possessor off (sic) as deviant, flawed, spoiled, or undesirable' (p. 14).

They state that once the stigma is assigned, a construct or theory may be developed to explain its existence. In order to do this certain criteria need to be met:

- the selection of a negative attribute;
- perceptions by others of the negative attribute;
- resultant widespread devaluation of the possessor, frequently including labelling and communication of the labels.

They cite Jones et al.'s (1984) six major dimensions that are particularly influential:

1 conceal ability;
2 course;
3 disruptiveness;
4 aesthetic qualities;
5 origin;
6 peril.

Kasperson et al. also state that risk amplification can occur with the release of a government report that provides new information. The presentation of the information to the general public creates an awareness of the risk, rather than personal experience. The media form a pivotal role in the dissemination of the new knowledge by 'framing' the risk with the use of metaphors, symbols and language, thus depicting and characterising the risk. Stigmatisation arising from risk-related attributes involves three stages:

1   The risk related attributes receive high visibility, particularly through communication processes, leading to perception and imagery of high riskiness, a process that we refer to as the social amplification of risk.

2   Marks are placed upon the person, place, technology or product to identify it as risky and therefore undesirable.

3   The social amplification of risk and marking alter the identity of the person, place, technology or product, thereby producing behavioural changes in those encountering the imagery and marking as well as those to whom they are directed.

Accompanying this process will often be a story or narrative that interprets the evolution of the stigma and assigns responsibility or blame for its presence. (p.19)

The framework describes how a trigger event leads to responses by information channels and may result in individual responses. The model also outlines how these responses produce ripple effects that over time may have consequences not only for an individual and their community but also for the society as a whole and possibly global impact.

Central to the framework is the concept of 'attenuation'. This relates to the extent to which individuals act or do not act on the perceived risk. It appears that the repeated amplification of a risk can result in individuals becoming used to the message and not acting on relevant advice to minimise the hazard.

The amplification of obesity as a global problem illustrates Kasperson et al.'s framework. The amplification of the risk from obesity has taken place at different times dependent on the country involved. North America has been aware of the issue for longer than European countries. The trigger factors will be varied; for example in Britain the publication of the National Audit Committee of the House of Commons Report on Obesity in 2001, prompted major media coverage. Emphasis was placed on both individuals and place. The *Sun* newspaper headed their coverage with the picture of the Union Jack and the caption 'Weight Britain' (February 2001). Deborah Lupton (2005) highlights a similar approach in Australia. Even in countries such as Taiwan obesity has come to the fore with headlines stating 'Big in Taiwan' (BBC, 1 September 2000) along with a picture of children undertaking a session of compulsory aerobics.

Once a problem has been amplified then the extent of the problem needs to be established. Kasperson et al. state that for action to be taken a perceived risk will go through a number of phases. Firstly, the risk is perceived, and then it is communicated via different sources of information. This will include both direct and indirect communication or be based on personal experience. Information channels which include individual senses, informal channels and professional information brokers will then come into play.

An example of how obesity issues can be communicated via informal sources is through the use of popular fiction or television programmes other than documentaries. Kyle Mills (2003) in his thriller *Smoke Screen* invents a character who works for a tobacco industry due to a trust agreement. In a fictional television debate about the health risk of smoking the character agrees that cigarettes are harmful but states they are not the most dangerous product that the company sells. When asked what it is he says, 'I would have to say those boxes of little doughnuts – you know, the ones with the powdered sugar on them' (p162). He goes on to state their contribution to diabetes and obesity. The doughnuts are then regularly included in the story line. At the end he gives up smoking but it is unclear whether he stops eating the doughnuts.

Direct action usually occurs when the risk is accepted at the level of social stations and individual stations. This gives the impetus to changes in institutional and social behaviour. This includes political action. What forms do these actions take and to what extent can the needs of individuals be met when approaching problems from a national or global perspective?

In relation to obesity, a number of approaches have been used. Some countries have acted by examining changes in the diet and establishing what is a healthy diet. Others have embarked on health campaigns that include provision of a wide range of information. This includes specialist websites: Singapore is one of these with an overall strategy that targets different groups. Their website includes a range of information, advice on diet and exercise including health diaries and games (Singapore Health Promotion Board Online 2005[1]). Other initiatives have focused on food in schools and education in relation to diet.

One of the issues is that obesity is being dealt with in different ways by different groups. Swinburn et al. (2005) suggest there is a need to provide evidence-based approaches to dealing with obesity. They note that public health measures and clinical measures usually have different foci. A plethora of information about the possible causes of obesity exists as does a range of material about what to do but little is evidence based. Swinburn et al. designed a decision-making framework for The International Obesity Taskforce which will enable an evidence-based approach to prevention of obesity.

The framework has five parts:

1   building a case for action on obesity;
2   identifying the contributing factors and points of intervention;
3   defining the range of opportunities for action;
4   evaluating potential interventions;
5   selecting a portfolio of specific policies, programmes and actions.

The aim of the framework is to provide strong research-based knowledge to ensure that policies and programmes introduced are achievable and sufficient to reduce obesity.

The portfolio mentioned above will include a range of policies and programmes which take into account stakeholders' needs and their judgement of the implications of these. The portfolio will therefore have a range of options and thus not fall into the one-size-fits-all trap.

Interventions will be assigned a level of 'promise' – high, medium or low. In some instances a number of low-level promises may be more effective than a high-level promise due to ease of implementation and sustainability. This takes into account the setting in which the policy or programme is being implemented and also the likelihood of adoption of individuals. They are also concerned with preventing stigmatisation.

Kwankam (2004) advocates the use of E-health in order to bridge the gap between what is known and what we do. E-health is defined as Internet and other forms of electronic information used for clinical, educational, research and administrative purposes. Effective dissemination of selective, targeted information can be beneficial in delivering health information to health professionals and lay people thus aiding the saving of lives. In order for the information to be effective it needs to be 'just-in-time', high quality and relevant. With changes in technology the information can be available for developing countries but needs to be multi-lingual. One criticism of this is that sensitivity to cultural differences may be difficult to achieve.

---

1   www.hpb.gov.sg/hpb/default.asp?pg_id=985

Bailey and Pang (2004) confirm this. They see that provision of information is important, but it is necessary to understand how information is used locally. They state that policy makers in developing countries prefer to use local research. Problem solving needs to build on the existing knowledge rather than solely on imported knowledge.

Ania Lichtarowicz (2004) reinforces this. Being large has been associated with wealth. In South Africa emphasis on becoming slim is not appropriate as this is the term used to describe victims of AIDS. Alternative approaches, therefore, have to be considered.

Kasperson et al. (2001) emphasises the difficulties in relation to trans-boundary risk. One of the reasons given for the growth of obesity in developing countries is the introduction of Western influences. Previous conflicts may influence reactions to measures being introduced and lead to attenuation of the risk. For example, North America can be seen as benefiting from the introduction of fast food to other countries and therefore may not be trusted if they lead plans to deal with the issue. Overcoming the need to ascribe blame to an individual, place or nation is therefore essential to enable action to be taken.

To what extent are these messages acted upon and in what way?

The messages regarding obesity are being received by individuals and groups and at some levels measures are being introduced to deal with the issue. The WHO Consultation on Obesity (June 1997) placed emphasis on strategies to prevent weight gain and obesity as this is more cost effective and easier than treating obesity once developed. They noted that measures to treat obesity have met with different degrees of success. One problem is that emphasis on weight loss has health consequences and it is doubtful that achieving a target weight is beneficial.

Obesity management therefore needs to cover a range of issues namely prevention of weight gain, weight maintenance, management of obesity comorbidities and weight loss. WHO suggest three levels of prevention:

- universal/public health prevention (directed at everyone in the population);
- selective prevention (directed at sub-groups of the population with an above average risk of developing obesity);
- targeted prevention (directed at high-risk individuals who may have a detectable amount of excess weight but who are not yet obese). (p. 167)

Adams and White (2005) express concern over the population approach to health promotion. If interventions have the effect intended and where the relationship between exposure and risk is continuously positive then population approaches are beneficial for all individuals in the population. However when a J curve occurs some individuals will be disadvantaged by population approaches. They use the example of obesity, in that although there is compelling evidence of health problems by concentrating in this area, underweight is also a cause of ill health and may be overlooked. They also cite recent research that shows an increase risk of death is associated in apparently healthy individuals with a BMI index of 18 and under compared to those with a BMI of between 20–22.

They highlight that all public health initiatives have the potential to cause harm as well as good. The harm is often seen as unavoidable and unimportant compared to the overall good. Public health approaches may put the message across, but it may not be the one received or not received by target audience. Rather than reducing obesity, an increase in underweight may occur. Poor patterns of eating may result as people become confused by conflicting information and advice. Some actions such as 'healthier school meals' may disadvantage those who are underweight or have a high metabolic rate through restricting portion size.

Assessment of public health initiatives have noted that although information is given this is not always acted on. Davison et al.'s (1992) concept of the apocryphal 'Uncle Norman' points to one explanation. Risk perception is based on the idea that Uncle Norman is still healthy despite following the unhealthy lifestyle being referred to.

Webb et al. (2002: 23) describe a number of blockage points which can act as barriers to effective health promotion.

- The receiver fails to see or hear the message.
- The message may not gain the attention of the target group.
- The message may not be understood by the receiver.
- The message may not be believed or if it is too complex and not reinforced, it may be forgotten.
- Behaviour change does not occur despite message being received and understood.
- Behaviour change occurs but does not result in improved health.

Kasperson et al.'s (op. cit.) concept of 'attenuation' confirms how actions in relation to risk may not occur. The different types of information and suggested approaches to the problem may lead to inaction as it becomes rhetoric rather than reality.

The rise in the incidence of obesity can be seen as predictable. Bazerman and Watkins (2004) postulate the concept of 'predictable surprises'. They suggest that often potential or actual risks are known but not acted on. They propose a number of cognitive biases that may be used, thus affecting perception of risk.

The first is that we create 'positive illusions' and therefore see the problem as sorting itself out. Secondly, we interpret the situation from our own viewpoint and not from that of others. They cite Kimberly Wade-Benzoni et al.'s work (1996) on pollution of the River Rhine. The Rhine flows through five different countries, all of which at some point contribute to pollution but at differing levels. The Rhine provides a range of services including a source of drinking water and fishing. The upstream countries have lower pollution than downstream due to the accumulated effect. Downstream countries which bore the brunt of the pollution were perceived to be the most interested in sorting the problem with emphasis on fair access to clean water, whilst upstream countries emphasis was seen to focus on the economic effects any actions would have.

This illustrates that any actions proposed to combat a risk may have to take into account a range of perspectives that include trans-national working and in some incidents global collaboration.

Another perceptual bias is that if we or someone close to us, have not experienced the problem, then we do not act on it. The other forms of bias are 'discounting the future' and 'maintaining the status quo' this means that short-term solutions or no actions are favoured rather than long term. All the above may mean that a risk may be identified but little or no actions may be taken.

Through looking at the literature in relation to other food risks, lessons can be learnt in relation to possible approaches. The incidence of human mercury contamination in the Amazon was initially thought to be the result of gold mining in the 1970s with the use of mercury to extract the gold and the subsequent pollution of the Amazon River. Ecological research carried out by a joint Brazilian and Canadian team (Johnson 2003) over a decade has established that although the mining contributed to the presence of mercury, agricultural practices have compounded the problem. Their findings illustrated the need to be open minded in the approach to understanding causation.

The case also highlights the complexity of risk and the different chain of events that lead from and to the physical manifestations of symptoms. The incidence of methyl mercury poisoning in Brasilia Legal led to the perception of a major health risk. Understanding of the mining practices and of how mercury is converted to methyl mercury led to examination of the water supply. Mercury is a naturally occurring substance which was deposited in the soil following volcanic activity centuries ago. The mercury evaporated into the air and was deposited in the soil via rainfall. The deposits became buried over time until agricultural changes occurred. Deforestation resulted in topsoil being washed away thus exposing the subsoil which is mercury rich. The mercury became washed into the water and converted to methyl mercury. This then entered the food chain resulting in high mercury levels in fish which were then eaten by humans. As other animals also eat fish then meat became another source of poisoning.

The research highlighted that levels of methyl mercury increased if fish that ate other fish were consumed. Herbivorous fish produced lower levels. Measures to address the problem included the use of posters to encourage eating the right type of fish, examination of the diet that identified foods which reduced the uptake of mercury, and identification of hot spots where the mercury was more concentrated resulted in management of the plant life in the river. However, although the measures addressed the problems in relation to diet and included the local community, this did not address the deforestation and soil erosion.

The continued deforestation has increased due to the change of farming to cattle ranching (CIFOR 2003). Some policies in Brazil appear to favour development rather than protection of the rainforest raising concerns in relation to global warming. However, other laws try to restrict the amount of damage but these are difficult to enforce. Other measures such as sustainable crops are also being advocated. In 2003, Brazil voted to save the 7 per cent remaining Atlantic rainforest from further development (Hay 2003).

Research carried out by Rahman et al. (2005) looked at the levels of arsenic contamination of groundwater in West Bengal, India, and the health impacts. What is interesting about the study is that although the scientific evidence is conclusive and there are visible signs of health problems in individuals, the measures that are available to prevent the problem (the use of arsenic-filtering devices, advice on depth of wells and so on) have not been taken on board by the local population. The research does not explore why this is.

Dale (2003) presents a case study in relation to pesticide poisoning in potato crops in Ecuador. Pesticides are used to control a number of pests which can blight the potato crop. Persistent use of toxic pesticides has continued despite known health problems, and lack of protective clothing and safety precautions have added to the risk.

Approaches to combat the problem had to address the interests of the farmers, the population and the agro-chemical industry. Schools were set up showing families how the chemicals transferred between people and in the homes. Farmers were able to experiment with different forms of pest control and using a combination of approaches were able to produce the same level of yield but at a reduced cost.

The use of safety equipment and measures to prevent the travelling of pesticides also contributed to a reduction in health problems. Pesticides are still used but this is being addressed at policy level and the more harmful pesticides are being prohibited. Agro-chemical companies have funded initiatives for health and safety training, resulting in a comprehensive information package being created for the local communities.

The above examples give guidance on what may be the best ways to approach health issues. However, emphasis is on dealing with existing problems rather than prevention.

Measures by a range of countries to ensure indigenous diets are maintained (where applicable) are worthy of consideration and evaluation. Control of outside influences with the growth of technology and changes in the infrastructure may, however, negate this.

The social amplification of risk framework, suggests that once the issue is in the public domain ripple effects will occur. However, these may take time to become visible as will the long-term impacts.

Some of the ripple effects already identified are the change in menu in many fast-food outlets. There have also been a mixture of reactions to obese people. The television media coverage including programmes such as *The Biggest Loser* and *Fat Camp* are examples of the-individual-has-the-problem approach. Others such as *Fat Friends* and sketches in *Little Britain* take a comic view of obesity. Others take a more medical approach. Others look at more extreme issues as in *Fat Girls and Feeders* (Channel 4, Britain). In the Unites States programmes such as *Fat Actress* and *Monique* take differing views but lead to the same conclusion in that big is not necessarily bad. Very few look at group issues.

The association of risk with food is an area that will continue to cause concern. Many of the measures being employed will relate to both common approaches and more culturally specific action. The concept of a portfolio approach advocated by The International Task Force on Obesity seems to be an appropriate response. One issue is that in order for any measures to be successful there has to be trust in the source.

Obesity is not a new condition. A number of approaches have been used with varied effects. It is difficult for many countries to take on the trappings of Western style economic development and still retain the possibly healthier lifestyle of their own culture.

Kasperson et al.'s framework forms a useful structure in which to examine risk amplification. It remains to be seen as to the long-term results of the present amplification of obesity or whether the range of information which can be confusing and contradictory will lead to attenuation.

The news media and governmental groups are frequently blamed for public overreaction to situations, such as the rising obesity rates around the world, an example of the social amplification of risk. A disconnect between public views regarding the consequences of obesity and necessary remedies on the one hand and expert opinion on these same questions on the other is a frequently identified consequence of this phenomenon. An examination of the ways in which scientific messages can distort public opinion or rationalise public policy suggests however that a more complex phenomenology is at work. Perceived risks can be attenuated as well as amplified, and many organisations besides the news media contribute to the shaping of public risk attitudes. Both social amplification and social attenuation of messages about the risks of obesity for example, evident in public responses to the television shows such as the *Celebrity Fat Club*, *The Biggest Loser* or Paul McKenna's *I Can Make You Slim*, continue to affect the debate about obesity worldwide.

Communicable diseases: cultural approaches to risk communication

There are much older approaches to risk communication that are embedded with the culture. For example, as the World War I was ending, a threat emerged that was even more lethal than the fighting that had killed so many young men in their prime. The influenza outbreak of 1918–19 claimed the lives of 20 to 40 million people worldwide. Strangely, for a disease that was so devastating, there is almost no cultural or artistic record of it. Two of the remaining pieces document the event with words rather than visual images. The first is a playground chant in which British children wove the effects of what they had witnessed into their daily games, so as they skipped rope they sang:

> I had a little bird
> Its name was Enza
> I opened the window
> And in-flu-enza.

It would be easy to dismiss this as purely a lighthearted childhood chant, but it captures the ability of this disease to affect anyone, with hardly a warning. The other piece is the novella *Pale Horse, Pale Rider* by Katherine Anne Porter. The story begins with Miranda's narrative in which she describes a fretful dream foreshadowing death as the first hint that she is becoming ill during the course of the influenza epidemic of 1917–18. The story takes the reader through a month of Miranda's life as a newspaper theatre columnist, a young single woman struggling with a relationship with a soldier about to be 'shipped over', and an observer of the World War I frenzy that engulfed America.

The final pages are made up of Miranda's intermittent delirious dreams and perceptions from the depth of her illness. She slowly recovers, only to learn that her fiancé soldier has succumbed to the same illness and dies suddenly and that the war has ended. In this tale is a treasure trove of personal insight into the war and the influenza epidemic along with descriptions of the response of the city to the epidemic. The close observation of the effect of illness on perceptions and reactions to the environment are instructive.

Within the last few years, influenza has become a rather hot topic which has been picked up within the arts. In Stephen King's novel and film *The Stand*, a 'superflu' virus wipes out much of the world's population. Terry Gilliam's 1997 film *Twelve Monkeys* also presents an apocalyptic vision. It tells the story of a society that has fled underground following the decimation of humankind by a flu-like plague. In 2004 the Public Broadcasting Service (PBS) aired an episode of *The American Experience* entitled 'Influenza: 1918'. This proved timely, since it followed on the heels of the bird flu in Hong Kong that captured the world's attention. Influenza has since made the covers of *Time* and *Rolling Stone* and been parodied in *Entertainment Weekly*.

Now that flu vaccines are dispensed at supermarkets and vehicle emissions testing sites in America, influenza has become a fixture of pop culture, much the way the common cold has been for years. But there remains a difference; we do not laugh at the thought of influenza, particularly avian flu, as the following passage illustrates.

Politics, fear and health risk communication: examples from avian flu and HIV/AIDS

According to Barzani (2006) the number of Kurdish siblings succumbing to the highly pathogenic form of avian influenza is on the rise:

> *This deadly pandemic (bird flu) recently detected in Kurdistan continues claiming the lives of many underprivileged and improvised [sic, impoverished] Kurdish citizens in Kurdistan (Southeastern Turkey). According to some complaints filed, most affected Kurdish victims are being turned down proper hospitalisation or medical attention for symptoms that suggest avian influenza. Preventive measures on behalf of Turkish health authorities and international intervention appear inadequate.*

> *Rumours abound that the spread of bird flu is part of the Turkish deliberate plot to multiply panic among Kurdish citizens, to mitigate their rural population (modern Turkification policy) and enforce a mandatory relocation into urban areas.*

In Papua rumours are also rife, inspiring conspiracies as illuminated in the following quote published by Butt (2005):

> *This is what I've heard: Since the problem of Free Papua arose, AIDS has come here so that Papuans die off. There were these fallen women [perempuan sundal] from Jayapura, well they [the Indonesian government] brought them all to Wamena. And those who want those women can have sex with them. And the women brought the disease with them.*

Butt informs us that according to widespread theorising among indigenous Papuans, 'lipstick girls' and 'fallen women' infected with HIV were introduced into Papua as part of an Indonesian programme aimed at eliminating indigenous people from the resource-rich province. Papuans have heard through media and gossip that the number of HIV and AIDS cases in the province are the highest per capita in Indonesia and that the province is on the verge of an epidemic. According to Butt, the core logic of Papuan theories about the causes for this links AIDS with political conditions of disempowerment and that such assertions are made by numerous Papuans from many places and walks of life.

   Both HIV/AIDS and influenza in our times have become major international political dilemmas. In the case of influenza the question is, how do we prepare ourselves for a potentially catastrophic pandemic without generating widespread public panic? In the case of HIV/AIDS the questions remains, how do we halt the spread of the disease, encourage compliance with precautionary measures, treat people with the disease and ensure they maintain their drug therapy to avoid drug resistance?

   Scholars have used the term 'rumour' to describe forms of talk to deal with, usually in a highly evocative symbolic manner, seemingly unrelated events. Taussig (1987) and Masquelier (2000) consider that these interpretations provide the means for people to make sense of political or economic conditions. Butt (2005) claims that in a number of societies, prostitutes and sexually transmitted diseases (STDs) have provided potent symbols in rumours of otherness, contagion, assault and invasion. Sexuality offers a salient marker of otherness while stigmatised prostitution particularly highlights external threats to communities (Jeffrey 2002; Stoler 2002). Treichler, for example, notes that in South Africa it is widely believed that AIDS enables control over the reproduction of blacks, a view that is also held by many Malawians (Hillier 1992 unpublished research). Similarly, inmates in American prisons cast AIDS as part of deliberate campaigns to exterminate communities of colour (Treichler 1999, 319).

Clearly, both AIDS and sex workers are particularly good to 'think with' as cultural categories for articulating power relations by oppressed groups. The oppositions between rumour and fact, on the one hand, and between emotional release and political analysis, on the other hand, fail to capture the complexity of people's discursive response to communicable diseases such as HIV/AIDS or avian flu.

Case study: sexual health

Charlotte Lapsansky of Breakthrough TV informs us that almost 85 per cent of HIV/AIDS infections in women result from sex with their husbands or primary partners. Yet, only 5 per cent of Indian women have comprehensive knowledge about ways to prevent HIV/AIDS. Women suffer various forms of violence all through their lives; HIV/AIDS has now added to these problems because women find it very difficult to negotiate safe sex or condom use, whether as sex workers, wives or girlfriends. In response, Breakthrough (www.breakthrough. tv/Campaign_detail.asp?cid=12), an international human rights organisation that uses media, education and pop culture to promote values of dignity, equality and justice, launched a multimedia campaign in an effort to bring public attention to the growing incidence of HIV/AIDS among women in India. The campaign uses television, radio, printed materials, cinema/theatres, educational forums and the Internet to promote equality within marriage and to encourage a deeper understanding of human rights issues in India. The aim is to enable women to negotiate condom use and other measures to protect themselves from HIV/AIDS and other infections.

The 'What Kind of Man Are You?' campaign promotes use of male condoms to prevent the spread of HIV/AIDS while addressing the gender inequality that leads to greater vulnerability of women with regard to HIV/AIDS. By using entertainment media, Breakthrough hopes to spark a discussion about difficult but pivotal issues like fidelity, protection from HIV/AIDS and communication within marriage.

The main communication approaches – it is hoped – will enable women to negotiate condom use and other measures to protect themselves from HIV/AIDS and other infections. What are intended to be sensitive yet tough/masculine campaign messages have been translated into six languages: Bengali, Hindi, English, Kannada, Tamil, Telegu and Marathi. The campaign also includes a music video featuring popular actors Mandira Bedi and Samir Soni.

The Breakthrough campaign also draws on in-person events to raise the issue of HIV/ AIDS from the point of view of women while also calling for male responsibility. Specifically, Breakthrough is conducting workshops and educational forums with students, homemakers, medical and legal professionals, and other groups on women's rights and HIV/AIDS to encourage a deeper understanding of human rights issues in India. Breakthrough states that the rates of HIV infection among women in India are steadily rising. Women account for around 40 per cent of documented cases of people living with HIV/AIDS. Of these, only 0.5 per cent of the women are sex workers. The biggest HIV/AIDS risk for many women and girls is heterosexual sex.

Of course sexual health is a very important topic but the messages also have an impact and consequences. Poonam Thapa thinks that positive sexual health messages change how we think about sexuality and have an impact on reducing risk.

Communicating risk in sexual health: a risky business?

WHY NOW?

Pleasure and desire for intimacy are forces for good. They play a major role in people's lives both personally and professionally. However, increasingly in modern life, time constraints can leave people de-prioritising the role of sexual play in the private domain. Sex is not the problem and yet it has become one.

More than 20 million people globally have died of AIDS-related diseases. At least twice that figure (40 million) live with HIV, and most of these are likely to die over the next decade. The most recent UNAIDS/WHO estimates show that, in 2004 alone, 4.9 million people were newly infected with HIV.[2] WHO estimates that 340 million new cases of syphilis, gonorrhoea, chlamydia and trichomoniasis occurred throughout the world in 1999 in men and women aged 15–49 years.[3]

It is disappointing that the global numbers of people infected continue to increase, despite the fact that prevention and protection strategies already exist and have been evolving for two decades. What is the missing link – could it be the absence of the erotic form, sensible pleasures and emotional safety in relationships with oneself and others? – as part and parcel of the concept that we know as 'safer sex' in the public and private sector?

What is at risk – could it be openness and honesty on both sides of the great divide between public sector and the commercial sex industry? We agree that 'pleasure needs cultivation, in the realm of sex nature requires culture' (Doniger and Kakar 2002) but in the search for the Holy Grail are we confusing ideals and myths with realities and options?

Look around you! Sex becomes a sensitive subject only when one is trying to have a serious discussion about it – this is a risk. The greatest risk of all, however, is that when it comes to truth and sex, we censure ourselves and each other around that professional table.

PLEASURE SEX IS SAFER SEX

Sex that is fun, feels good and is exciting can still be safe, and safer sex brings relaxation that can allow better enjoyment. Knowing how to have and talk about good sex allows more opportunities to have safer sex. Because protected sex is perceived as rarely fun and fun sex is rarely safe, relevant programmes in sexual and reproductive health and rights have become a means for damage control rather than one promoting practical solutions for modern times. Simultaneously through the discovery and development of sexual pleasure, greater overall self-confidence and self-esteem can be gained, which in turn leads to a greater ability to make empowered decisions around safer sex.

The health-based discussions of sex brought by the HIV/AIDS epidemic have, however, meant that sex is now openly (although negatively) discussed in areas where this was previously impossible. This paves the way for a sex-positive message to be sensitively slipstreamed into

---

2   'Around the World', Avert, www.avert.org/aroundworld.htm.
3   1999 data has been used as WHO has no publication after this date on the subject of sexually transmitted infections worldwide.

even the most reticent of cultures, resulting in more successful safer-sex programming and improved sexual health.

COMMUNICATING RISK THROUGH PLEASURE

A recent exercise to create a global map[4] of sex-positive and pleasure promotion initiatives indicates that many practitioners are using the obvious benefits of promoting sexual pleasure to motivate safer sex. A few health promotion agencies and programmes have linked enhancement of pleasure as a result of using their condoms. Commercial condom marketing often uses images of enhanced pleasure, and recently has started promoting condoms with sexual lubricant for added pleasure.[5]

The female condom has also been promoted in many countries as a pleasure-enhancing device due to increased sensitivity and heat conduction properties. The Society for Women and AIDS in Senegal[6] promoted the female condom as an erotic accessory – to great programmatic success.

A recent initiative in India[7] uses the texts of the *Kama Sutra* to enable sex workers to make the clients happy without penetrative sex. Sexual interest can be maintained by eroticisation of putting on male condoms or insertion of female ones, as well as non-penetrative sex. Christian organisations in Southern Africa have offered sex-positive marriage counselling to reduce infidelity.[8]

The recent satellite session at the Bangkok AIDS conference ('Can we only have safer sex if we know how to have good sex?') hosted by The Pleasure Project confirmed the commitment and enthusiasm for pleasure-promoting approaches to safer sex by health organisations and the need to enhance skills for sex educators to discuss pleasure and desire.

A subsequent programme of training for Cambodian and Vietnamese sex educators for CARE International created an environment of skills enhancement for education in good and safer sex. Sex educators working with young people learnt skills that allowed them to relate more openly with vulnerable young people and provide relevant services. The training illustrated that sexual health trainers can be enabled to discuss sex and pleasure.[9]

MORAL OF THE STORY

The communication of risk, as much as it may be a matter of life and death, is about education and learning. Nonetheless, we must go beyond the classroom attitude and face the reality of consumerism governed by the fancy of getting things 'here and now.' The marketplace is a good example of the nature of modern man and woman – chasing desires and furthering pleasure in all forms – so why should it be any different in the bedroom?

Ten golden rules for sex educators to reduce sexual health risk are outlined below:

---

4   Global Mapping of Pleasure – The Pleasure Project, www.the-pleasure-project.org, Dec 2004 – global database of any work in the sexual health field that has utilised pleasure to motivate safer sex.
5   As in the above second case study.
6   'Eroticizing the Female Condom, How To Increase Usage'. Reference No 350823, ICASA African AIDS Conference, July 2003.
7   'Kamasutra' invites UN attraction, AIDS-INDIA (19 October 2003).
8   Global Mapping of Pleasure (as above) Case Study 1.
9   Report of three-day training course on 'Sex, Safer Sex & Pleasure' facilitated by The Pleasure Project for CARE International & CARE, Cambodia, Phnom Penh, 14–16 December 2004.

- Communicate safety but allow people to conclude their own risk.
- Be sex-positive especially in the face of moral order and institutional anxieties.
- Talk about sex in real time – the here and now.
- Weave your own life into any sexual dialogue – people will trust you more.
- Remember pleasurable sex is about gravitas, generosity and heart.
- Always keep in mind that sexual health is about happiness first and foremost – happy people make better decisions.
- Stop social exclusion, stigma and taboo attached to words like pleasure, desire, emotions, affection, intimacy, sexuality, seduction, fantasy, prowess and allure, to name a few in public discourses around sexual and reproductive health.
- Connect with the 'other sector' (public with private and vice versa) using real-life situations and embellishment – an invitation to come into each others' space.
- Let the commercial sex industry know they can create value around sexual health and human rights and still turn a profit.
- Schools need to begin recruiting external expertise in sexuality education – trainers who come with real-life experience. It would certainly make amends to the current situation of having the embarrassment of opening up sexually to the biology or physical education teacher.

Conclusion

In this chapter we have travelled along a road that has taken us from concepts of social amplification of risk as applied to obesity, briefly alluded to toxic contamination of our food supply, explored how culture, as exemplified in the arts and nursery rhymes, rumour and gossip all play a part in the complex process of health risk communication. We have seen how risk messages can carry cultural and political ideals that may well distort and divert normal human interactions in basic pleasures such as sex.

Health risk communication is not simple: it is bound up in politics and in commercial and personal interests. In the next chapter, Andy Stevens begins to uncover why young people choose to take up risky behaviours.

7 Fast Cars and Cool Cigarettes – Resilience of Risky Behaviour in Young People
by Andy Stevens

Hazardous behaviour has been an essential element of teenage lifestyles, at least since the 1950s. Films such as *Rebel Without a Cause* (1955) include violence, sexual experimentation, drinking, smoking and reckless driving. Given my current lifestyle, my co-authors would be amused by the fact that my own teenage years involved all these elements (some more than others) and it has to be acknowledged that most teenagers of all eras experiment with, rather than habitually adopt, risky lifestyles. Teenagers in the twenty-first century exhibit the same behaviours with probably the same frequency, but the world has changed. There are fewer constraints (economic and social) on teenagers' decisions in Western societies (more so elsewhere for young people, particularly female) but there are also greater dangers, particularly HIV/AIDS, and there is more information available on dangers to health. So why do teenagers decide to take up such risky behaviours? Let us consider two behaviours with different forms of risk – smoking and reckless driving.

Smoking

Demographically, one of the riskiest decisions a young person can take is to start smoking. Tobacco smoking is a high-risk habit which kills about half of those who regularly practice it. In 2004, on average, 23 per cent of British men and women aged 16 or more were cigarette smokers; this proportion was higher for smokers under 25 years (25 per cent of women and 31 per cent of men), but there has been an overall decline in teenage smoking since 1995 (36 per cent and 39 per cent, respectively) (Lader and Goddard 2005). An earlier Britain, 82 per cent of adult smokers started regular smoking in their teens or earlier (DoH 1998). There are about 114 000 smoking-related deaths each year in Britain; five times more deaths than the combined results of road and other accidents, drugs, murder, manslaughter, suicides and HIV infection (www.ash.org.uk). An estimated global total of 4.9 million premature deaths were due to tobacco smoking in 2000, with a projected figure of 9 million deaths by 2020. While smoking rates decline in developed countries, rates are rapidly rising in the developing world and will account for nearly 78 per cent of the 2020 death total (Shafey et al. 2003).

Common assumptions for the causes of young people taking up smoking are that they are ignorant of the risks or that that it is a part of adolescent rebelliousness. While fatal effects of smoking are obviously not immediate, other effects, especially on respiration are quickly evident. Most smoking prevention campaigns focus on giving information, but young people in Britain are not ill-informed. Apart from warnings on cigarette packs and television of the risks, they receive and retain information given to them at school. When asked, 99 per cent of teenagers agreed that smoking causes lung cancer, and 68 per cent recalled having lessons on smoking the previous year (DoH 1998). A Chinese study found that teenagers were also well aware of the dangers of smoking (Yang et al. 2004). This confirmed the WHO Global Youth Tobacco Survey (GYTS 2002) finding that 83 per cent of students aged 13–15 years of age in Guangdong, China, knew of the dangers of smoking. Research on social patterns of take-up of smoking suggests that for teenagers who smoke, this is an act of social conformity not rebellion.

Comparative smoking frequencies

Frequency of smoking in populations varies around the world. More wealthy countries tend to have lower rates. Smoking frequency for men was at a peak of 82 per cent in 1948 and women peaked at 45 per cent in 1966 in the United Kingdom, but more recently, about a quarter of adults (of both sexes) smoke which is similar to countries such as the United States, Canada, Australia and the Netherlands. Sweden has a lower rate and atypically has a lower rate for men than women (17 per cent and 22 per cent). European countries with higher rates such as France (39 per cent and 27 per cent), Germany (43 per cent and 30 per cent) and Hungary (44 per cent and 27 per cent) show the more common higher frequency for men. Countries with non-European-based cultures vary considerably in tobacco consumption, but generally reflect cultural differences, particularly gender. Low consumers such as Nigeria (15 per cent and 2 per cent), Iran (25 per cent and 5 per cent) and Singapore (27 per cent and 3 per cent) and the very high consumers such as the Philippines (75 per cent and 18 per cent), Kenya (67 per cent and 32 per cent), China (63 per cent and 4 per cent) and Japan (53 per cent and 31 per cent) indicate cultural differences in attitudes to women smoking are a stronger influence on frequency than national economic development (figures from Corrao et al. 2000). Cigarette tar content in many Asian countries is often much higher than the European regulation of 12 mg. Highest frequencies of male smoking is closely correlated to high rates of national economic growth (Stevens and Caan forthcoming). Current highest frequency countries have not necessarily reached their peak in consumption (Yang et al. 2004).

Differences can also be found in smoking frequency between classes and ethnic groups within countries. Men and women in professional jobs smoke much less than those in unskilled manual jobs (16 per cent and 29 per cent for men and 18 per cent and 29 per cent for women, respectively) in the UK (Lader and Goddard 2005). Bangladeshi, Irish and Black Caribbean males have a higher-than-average rate of smoking, but other Asian males and all ethnic minority women have less than average rates (JHSU 2001). African American males also have the highest smoking rates in the United States (Nevid 2000); this rate is about 50 per cent (Juon et al. 2002).

Smoking initiation

The frequency of early-onset smoking is not surprisingly linked to other risky or socially disruptive behaviour by young people in most juvenile smoking research. Risk of nicotine addiction increases with frequency of experimentation by young people.

> *Addiction to nicotine is far more common than addiction to cocaine and the rate of graduation from occasional use to addictive levels of intake is highest for nicotine in the form of cigarettes. Depending upon the definition used for occasional use, 33–90 per cent of occasional users escalate to become daily smokers.*
>
> (RCP 2000 4.4)

The speed of addiction is unpredictable for teenagers, but problems of addiction are evident in adolescent cultures, as 72 per cent of smokers under 15 years old in one study have tried to give up (Higgins 1999). However, decisions to take up smoking cannot be just individual ones, or even subcultural, given the wide variations in smoking frequencies worldwide.

The WHO Global Youth Tobacco Survey (GYTS 2002) of 13 to 15 year olds gives a picture of the variation between cultures of 43 countries identified. Half of those smoking in India started before they were 10 years old. The highest rate of habitual smokers was found in Chile (39.6 per cent), but the lowest was in Goa, India (0.5 per cent). Over a third of students were current smokers in six sites (three in Chile, Moscow, Kiev, and the Northern Mariana Islands). Moscow, had one of the highest rates of current cigarette smoking (33.4 per cent), but with the least likely to smoke at home (4.8 per cent). Reasons for smoking were asked and responses varied widely, but boys who smoked were considered more socially astute and attractive than girls. Overall, 68.4 per cent of smokers wanted to stop – 86.9 per cent in China, which had the highest frequency of smokers in the study (GYTS 2002). The strongest predictor of regular smoking in China is peer influence in an under-20s study (Yang et al. 2004). This suggests that generalisations from local research into smoking should be treated with caution. Regional and national variations suggest complex attitudes to smoking habits within cultures.

Most research tends to be in European-based cultures and this strongly suggests that smoking initiation is socially mediated by both parents and peers. Smoking habits tend to run in families, which suggests both biological and social influences by parents. A Dutch study of primary schoolchildren (mean 11 years old) suggests that social pressures were less evident with younger children than adolescents, but that 28 per cent had experimented and nearly 8 per cent were regular smokers (Ausems et al. 2003). Fagan replicates numerous other studies of teenagers which suggest that parents' education, social class level and parental smoking habits are significant but associated influences, but additionally that parental attachment, particularly maternal aspirations for their child are significant (Fagan et al. 2005). Parents who had quit smoking reduce that risk of their offspring smoking, but this was still higher than parents who had never smoked (Bricker et al. 2003). Simon-Morton suggests that children engaged with friends with problem behaviour including smoking were less likely to smoke themselves if their parents were more involved with their lives irrespective of family background or race (Simmons-Morton 2003). A study of African-American teenagers shows that they develop smoking habits later than their white peers, but smoking frequency overtakes that of young white adults (Juon et al. 2002).

Female smoking is becoming more frequent in some developed countries such as New Zealand, Sweden and Norway, despite good health systems and information on the particular dangers of smoking during pregnancy. British teenage women are not yet as regular smokers as males – on most annual statistical returns young males predominate very slightly (Lader and Goddard 2005), even in regular smokers under 15 years old (Becher in Boreham and Shaw 2001). An Australian study of teenage girls indicates the importance of peers in female smoking take-up (Snow and Bruce 2003). A Dutch study indicates that females experiment with smoking later, but more rapidly become regular smokers (Galanti et al. 2001).

Smoking in advertising and media

It should not be assumed that advertising and mass media do not influence young potential smokers despite research clearly indicating the primary influence of family and friends on decisions to experiment and the take-up of cigarette smoking by children. This influence is difficult to quantify especially in European countries where there are now advertising restrictions regarding tobacco, although in many areas of the world advertising and promotion remain poorly regulated. TV smoking adverts were banned in the United States in 1965 and in the United Kingdom in 1971. In 1998 a European Union Directive banning all tobacco advertising phases out advertising, sponsorship and promotion in a staged phase-out by 2006. The WHO 192 Member States unanimously adopted the world's first public health treaty, the WHO Framework Convention on Tobacco Control in 2003. Smoking has also been banned in public places in countries as diverse as Ireland, Italy, Norway, Tanzania, Cuba, South Africa and parts of the Unites States, and will be in the United Kingdom by 2007. Business reports suggest that profits are little affected due to high profit margins (approximately 46 per cent in the UK) and increasing markets in Africa, Southeast Asia, and Eastern Europe with the takeover of the smaller, localized brands by the international companies (Business Week Online 19 January 2005). It is reasonable to suggest that tobacco companies would not invest such large sums on advertising and promotions such as sports events ($5.5 billion per annum, http:// tobaccofreekids.org) if this was not effective in increasing consumption. Tobacco companies still pay large placement fees to have their brands incorporated directly in films, resulting in smoking appearing in 2002 movies about as often as in 1950 movies, even though smoking was twice as prevalent in 1950 (Glantz et al. 2004).

Severe curtailment of the promotion of tobacco consumption does not in itself significantly reduce consumption. Despite the research evidence, smoking is still widely socially tolerated and tobacco is legally regulated less than cocaine or marijuana despite its more damaging effects. The intensity of marketing cigarettes over the past century has embedded the smoking habit within the cultures of the world. The tobacco genie is out of the bottle (or packet) and society has not properly addressed how it should be dealt with.

Smoking was considered a luxury until the beginning of the twentieth century, which marked the development of mass production of cheap cigarettes with rapid rises in consumption. Cigarette design and packaging were engineered to encourage new smokers, and advertising was targeted towards young people to take up the habit through cheaper packaging and promotional innovations such as cigarette cards (Lock et al. 1998). A policy of targeting young people has continued to be quite current practice, and a survey of advertising agencies in the United States shows that advertisers believe that tobacco advertising influences children's attitudes to smoking (82 per cent) and that tobacco advertising targets non-smoking teenagers. Release of tobacco company internal documents during recent legal actions in the United States provided evidence that a number of measures have been taken by them to increase sales by targeting young non-smokers, even as young as five years old. The details of the survey and these memoranda are now publicised on anti-smoking websites (for example http://tobaccofreekids.org). Colourful packaging of chewing tobacco products (gutka) and sweet-flavoured thin unfiltered cigarettes (bidis) are clearly designed to attract Asian children who have still found them easily available in some areas of the United Kingdom and United States (www.ash.org.uk; Factsheet 26). These mechanisms, together with advertising, promotions and free distribution of cigarettes, are more widespread in areas of the world less regulated.

Images of smoking in photography, film and television during the twentieth century have tended to imbue positive smoking with semiotic meanings, such as refinement, sophistication, intelligence and maturity. Mid-century gangster and war movies associate smoking with strong character, masculinity and comradeship. Depictions of professors, senior political figures and bank managers (who are usually male) tend to reinforce intelligence and respectability with pipe smoking. Iconic images of classic movie stars, such as Humphrey Bogart, Bette Davies, and John Wayne often feature smoking. Smoking is also iconically associated with romance – smoke trails caught by light in nightclubs or 'a cigarette that bears lipstick traces' ('These Foolish Things' – originally a French song) are examples. Tinkler's study of twentieth-century images of women's smoking indicates that for most of the century women smokers were invariably presented as young, modern and middle/upper class. One of the earliest negative images that she identifies is from 1970 – 'Give tobacco the brush-off', featuring an old, unattractive, working-class woman in a headscarf, which is actually an advert for toothbrushes (Tinkler 2003).

The re-presentation of these positive images of smoking in modern mass-media, including transfer to new media such as video games, is useful to modern media production, specifically because of the inherited cultural associations with smoking reinforced during the last century. Smoking provides a useful visual cue to indicate character maturity or a plot device to visually indicate internal thoughts. Guidelines are often given to television producers to confine depiction of smoking to programmes after a watershed period (9pm in the United Kingdom), or restrict it to films with mainly adult audiences. These guidelines change to reflect public attitudes. For example, BBC guidelines have recently changed from a position of balance (in 2005) towards restricted depiction of smoking:

> The acceptability of common forms of social behaviour like smoking or drinking tends to alter over time. There is a difficult balance to be struck by programme makers between the danger of encouraging potentially damaging habits, particularly amongst the young, and the need to reflect the range of public attitudes and behaviour realistically.
>
> In both drama and factual programmes, there are cases where smoking is essential to a character or story. But in general programmes, such as a studio debate, smoking is likely to be objectionable. Contributors can be reminded of such issues before recording begins.
>
> (www.bbc.co.uk/info/policies/producer_guides/text/
> section3.shtml; accessed March 2005)

Under these restrictions the essential-to-the-plot argument in practice offers very little restriction after the watershed. While smoking is rarely depicted in bars in BBC pre-watershed soap operas like *Eastenders*, it appeared to be necessary to the plot in the same type of scenes after the watershed, for example in *Hustle* (a light drama broadcast at 9pm in 2005).

Guidelines in 2006 avoid the essential-to-character argument for 'reflecting public attitudes and behaviour', but they are now clearly banning smoking in studio debates and chat shows and to avoid any positive associations with smoking where under-18s are likely to be watching – irrespective of the watershed (www.bbc.co.uk/guidelines/editorialguidelines; Section 8).

Public broadcasters to an extent passively reinforce traditional preconceptions about smoking through rescreening older programmes, but it is more difficult for commercial broadcasters in some countries who are more vulnerable to indirect tobacco company influence to place smoking products. Media depictions of smoking, at the least, passively inform young people about the importance of smoking in modern culture. Nevertheless, smoking is now mainly a habit of the young, including females in developed countries, although it remains largely a male practice in Africa and South Asia. Smoking is still fashionable, due to the reinterpretation of traditional imagery in current settings by visual mass-media – with little direct promotion by tobacco companies.

The use of mass-media campaigns to reduce smoking by young people has inherent difficulties. First, there are insufficient resources to challenge the current attitudes given the cultural position of smoking. Second, information is better delivered in schools and has been shown to be ineffective. Third, the most effective appeals tend to use fear as a cue to action. While death by cancer, amputation, severe respiratory and heart disease are frightening consequences of smoking, none of these consequences are as immediate to teenagers, in contrast to the effects of dangerous driving or failure to use car seatbelts (Delaney et al. 2004).

Governments consistently under-invest in anti-smoking measures. The UK Government has reluctantly agreed to ban public smoking, but does impose the highest tobacco excise in Europe. Nevertheless, current taxation does not cover the immediate social costs. The UK Government receives £8055 million in tobacco duty, but spends £71 million on trying to help people stop (£30 million on anti-smoking education, and the rest on smokers' cessation programmes) (www.ash.org.uk). Most anti-smoking advertising attracts government funding (Cancer Fund and Action for Smoking and Health), but this is funded indirectly and is targeted towards adults, as this is most effective. The misperception that health costs for smokers are less because they die younger has been raised in the press, but this has been promoted by Philip Morris and other tobacco companies (Rasmussen et al. 2004). Economically developing countries need greater anti-smoking measures but have even less funds for public health measures. The Philippines and India imposed advertising and tobacco control legislation in 2003, but tobacco companies have established large informal promotion systems in both countries. China has more recently banned further tobacco production factories and imposed higher tobacco taxation (February 2006), but it has the world's largest tobacco production, high rates of male consumption and the cheapest cigarettes in the world.

Smoking prevention programmes

There has been extensive research into the effectiveness of interventions to prevent or reduce frequency of smoking in young people. Thomas (2002) undertook a systematic review of 76 American and European randomised control trials evaluating school-based prevention programmes, but the overall conclusions were that there were few that showed any significance in prevention of smoking in young people. The nine evaluations of prevention programmes based on information-giving produced no significant results. The remaining studies involved social interventions, including building social competence, and using social influences, either in the classroom or in combination with the family or local community. Some studies (although few) suggested that there was some short-term positive influence in the reduction in take-up of smoking, and with these there is no evidence suggesting positive results were sustained. Research on the Hutchinson Smoking Prevention Project in the United States, a social influences project which ran for 15 years, failed to find a significant effect on smoking behaviour. Thomas was concerned that such programmes, which make heavy demands on teacher time, seem to have little long-term value. Some of these studies actually involved smoking cessation elements as well as prevention, which suggests that cessation programmes, that are quite effective with adults, are less successful with young people. A smaller review of 17 community interventions (some also used in the Thomas study) came to similar conclusions that most interventions had little discernible effects (Snowden et al. 2003). All of these studies relate to European-based cultures, but equally there is no indication that similar programmes in other cultures would have any better chances of success.

Smoking cessation programmes undertaken by adults appear to achieve much higher levels of success than intervention programmes with young people involving smoking cessation elements. In 2001/2 adult cessation programmes in the United Kingdom reported a 53 per cent success (over a month), but nicotine replacement (NRT) and/or bupropion was usually provided as part of the programme (84 per cent) (DoH 2002). Reviews of studies have demonstrated the effectiveness of NRT for cessation (for example Silagy et al. 2004). Chemical treatment for nicotine dependency appears to be a decisive element in cessation. However, NRT is not usually approved under the NHS as a treatment for those under 18 years.

Driving

Although reckless driving is not as big a killer as smoking-related disease, it kills more young people. It is also more visibly dangerous than smoking to teenagers because its effects are more immediate. Young drivers have a higher risk of involvement in road accidents and injury than other drivers, particularly crashes involving single vehicles, crashes on curves, night-time accidents and when driving at excessive speed (MacDonald 1994). Road accidents are the commonest cause of death for people under the age of 25 years in the United States, Canada and the European Union. In 1999, a UK report indicated that although 17 to 20 year olds held 11 per cent of licences they were involved in 25 per cent of fatal/serious accidents and that young male drivers (17–20 years old) had ten times more fatalities than mature drivers (34–50 years old) (DfT 2002). There were 7 353 fatalities due to drivers under 20 years old in the United States in 2003 (*Washington Post*, 9 September 2004).

Despite public concern over these figures, fatalities in these countries are comparatively low to those of the developing world. The highly motorised countries (HMCs) such as the United States, Canada, Western Europe and Japan) own 60 per cent of the cars, but have only 14 per cent of the global fatalities. Overall world road-fatality estimates are of around a million per annum (1.2 million in 2004 according to WHO), with around 30 million or more people injured. In a study of 43 countries, the highest individual fatality rates occur in some African countries, but over half the global fatalities occur in the Asia-Pacific region. While in HMCs rates have been falling over the past two decades, in developing countries they are rising in the Asia-Pacific region (by about 40 per cent between 1987 and 1995) (www.factbook.

net/EGRF_Summary.htm). This is a probable underestimate given a higher level of under-reporting in developing countries, particularly of non-fatal accidents. Global comparisons of driver behaviour and accident rates are difficult because of other variable factors relating to car design and condition and quality of roads. It would be sensible to infer that higher regulation of driving and better testing of vehicles and drivers are also likely to reduce accident levels in HMCs.

Research has variously suggested that increased risk of accidents by young drivers is due to:

- inexperience and poor driving skills;
- psychological factors (deliberate risk-taking, positive stress seeking, developmental immaturity);
- unsafe driving (speeding, racing, influenced by drink/drugs);
- poor estimates of ability and risk.

Driver liability to road accidents decreases with age and experience in both male and female drivers in the United Kingdom (Maycock in DfT 2002) and the United States (Mayhew et al. 2000). Speeding is the most common offence for young drivers, and there is a higher frequency of accidents in darkness. This is attributed to both inexperience and attitude. Night-driving can be correlated to alcohol consumption (in males of all ages) and recreational driving. Young people are particularly vulnerable to the effects of alcohol. Legal limits for drivers vary considerably between countries. England has one of the highest limits and under-21s account for 10 per cent of drink-driver convictions. However, male manual workers in their mid-20s and older male professionals are higher risk offenders (IAS 2005).

Attitudinal factors also affect young drivers' behaviour. Driving is considered to be fun, challenging, exciting, a way of testing themselves, and a way of showing off, rather than as comfortable and effective transport. Young drivers are influenced by the time and day of the week, but also passengers. Males will driver slower with older people and with peers who are female, than male peer passengers (Doherty et al. 1998). Restrictions on young drivers carrying peers reduces accidents (Cooper et al. 2005). Males with the highest rated self-confidence in driving and highest disposition for risk-taking were most likely to be repeated excessive speeders (Palmara and Stevenson 2003). A study of 17-year-old drivers in Western Australia showed that 66 per cent had speeding convictions in the first 36 months of driving. Conviction rates were highest in the second year (mainly minor infringements), but excessive speeding was highest in the first year of driving. A distinction has to be made between reckless and poor or novice driving. Some young drivers often have a 'test-pilot attitude', that is to consider the line between skilful and reckless driving to be more precise than it actually is, and therefore have insufficient safety margins (Clarke et al., in DfT 2002). Australian women drivers are more likely than males to be admitted to hospital as a result of a road crash. A survey of these drivers indicates that young women are more likely to be assertive, impatient or aggressive in their driving, but that lapses in concentration was the commonest causes of accidents (Dobson et al. 2000).

There is an interesting difference between car driving and motorcycling demographics. Statistics from the United Kingdom indicate that there has been a steady rise in casualties in older adults (25 to 59 years old), whereas accidents involving older and younger ages have declined (Department for Transport (DfT) 2004). Motorcycling has become a luxury pursuit, and those who use bikes for such purposes have more powerful machines and riskier attitudes to speed and drink-driving (DfT 2004). This suggests similarities in attitudes to younger car speeding drivers.

Unskilled car driving and inexperience which are commonest in novice drivers have been addressed by improvements in driver training and testing, legal restrictions on road use and other safety measures such as seat-belt laws, differential speed limits, that have been demonstrated as effective in reducing accidents for all drivers. Prior to belt laws, US wearing rates remained fairly constant for many years at about 14 per cent. After the passage of belt laws, rates increased over many years to 75 per cent by 2002. Two meta-analyses of road safety mass-media campaigns (including campaigns targeting young drivers) in HMCs suggested that they have a higher effect after the campaign than during it (on average 7.5 per cent to 8 per cent effect during and 14.8 per cent effect after in reducing crashes). Campaigns relating to alcohol and speeding were more effective and emotional rather than informational messages are likely to work best (Delaney et al. 2004).

Improvements in car safety technology, such as improved braking and crash cell design, have a negative correlation with increasing speed and numbers of accidents. Wilde (1994) considers individuals do not minimise levels of risk, but rather optimise benefits from risky behaviour according to environmental conditions to a 'target level of risk'. A state of equilibrium – 'risk homeostasis' – is maintained between risk-taking behaviour and the magnitude of loss due to accidents, which is only adjusted when there is a change in the target level of risk. Reckless drivers' target levels of risk are higher as they consider the particular benefits from risky driving (such as positive sensations from fast driving, gaining time or increased mobility) to be more valued than the costs of dangerous driving (fines, imprisonment, death), and the valuation of safer alternatives. Improvements in vehicle safety or better roads reduce the costs of risk to an individual, and thus increases their tolerance of risk.

Cultural context of teenage driving

Access to cars by teenagers varies between HMCs, but is usually only available to the most mature teenagers. The minimum legal age for driving varies normally between 17 and 18 years, but the lowest is in the United States, Canada, South Australia and New Zealand at 16 years. US states have their own regulations (including graduated licensing (Williams 2000)), but in some a learner/provisional licence can be obtained at 14 years. There are increasing calls for raising driving ages (*USA Today*, 3 February 2005). Car driving is also more accessible to young teenage Americans due to cars and fuel being lightly taxed and therefore driving is relatively cheap and generally preferred to public transport. Car ownership in America is therefore more often an essential element of mid-teen culture, than in many other countries. Arnett (2002) considers a crash rate 50 per cent higher for 16–17-year-olds, than 18–19-year-olds in the United States is a developmental or immaturity issue. A positive relationship with parents in a similar way moderates risky behaviour, but 'they spend more time in cars with friends and use their cars more for purposes that promote their social interactions, but are inimical to safe driving'.

Car driving has greater cultural significance for American teenagers, than most other cultures, an essential element of rite-of-passage teen movies, and from the 1950s in pop songs (for example by the Beach Boys or Chuck Berry). Traditional cultural images of the car (largely featuring white people) represent freedom and independence, and are situated in non-urban settings (drive-in, the beach, deserts and the open road), which are often features of advertising of new cars, which also invoke these feelings in older people who can afford them. Car advertising is primarily directed to post-teenage markets. However, there are other media images directed at young people (film and video games), which have a strong association with reckless driving. These images are located traditionally in film. VaRaces, a website dedicated to car chase films lists over 500 movies (www.varaces.com). A brief survey of current driving video games suggests that there are over 330 racing games on the market (most car, but also bikes and speed boats (www.gamespot.com). Some of these games feature racetracks or rallying, but others such as the popular *Grand Theft Auto* series feature realistic normal urban settings. Levels of speed and manoeuvring are managed by the operator. Children, too young to drive, may develop reckless attitudes to driving which may be transferred to their driving when older. Recent car chase films such as the remake *Gone in Sixty Seconds* (2001) and *The Fast and the Furious* (2001) have higher speed and crashes more like that of the interactive video game experience.

Association between car racing media and reckless driving, difficult to establish scientifically, has been present in news media 'folk-devil' representations of young car thieves in the United Kingdom and the United States, similar to the car-based hooligans or 'hoons' in Australia, as a threat to society.

A University of Western Sydney research programme looked at this 'hoon phenomenon' and the psychological influences of the media on such behaviour. The report presents the findings of a study of young people's reception of car advertisements and driver safety campaigns. It aimed to situate this reception within a socio-cultural context, by linking participants' responses to broader driving practices, attitudes and cultural meanings (Sofoulis et al. 2005). The findings confirmed that:

- Television was the most used medium, watched by 78 per cent of respondents (mainly between 6pm and midnight) followed by radio at 68 per cent (where usage peaked at morning drive time, and again in the late afternoon).

- Forty-one percent of respondents consumed magazines, almost two-thirds of which were car magazines, while billboards and the Internet were noted by over 30 per cent of respondents.

- There was high recall of messages about cars and driving from a wide range of sources, though film examples cited were mainly those featuring car culture, chases and racing.

- There was also high recall of both television and radio messages about road safety.

- While 90 per cent of respondents had played car racing video, computer or arcade games in younger years, only 11 per cent listed 'games' as part of their current media consumption.

The findings from the focus groups confirmed Sofoulis's (2003) earlier findings that the affective dimensions associated with speed correspond to the scenarios offered in a wide variety of car advertisements – escape, odyssey, conquests and cruising which capture key social values of freedom, autonomy and control.

Conclusions

Risky behaviour by young people elicits a greater response when that threat is immediate and personal, not only to young people, but others in society. Road accidents involving young drivers are no doubt too high, but are less due to recklessness in most of the world, than to poor road and vehicle conditions, driver instruction and regulation. Road deaths of young people in developed countries are particularly high because of the relative absence of other killers such as war, poverty and disease. Smoking kills in greater numbers eventually, but is a slower killer. Despite concerns about passive smoking and pregnancy, it is generally viewed as a threat to the individual. The duty of society in the case of smoking is merely to inform, but in the case of road safety to regulate.

Most people have experimented with drugs, such as tobacco, or broken speed limits and committed other road safety infringements, and are mostly likely to have done so during their youth. The riskiness of such behaviour appears to be less of an inhibiting factor on young people, but most of these actions are still within apparently safe boundaries. This is less obvious with smoking than road safety. Cultural associations of smoking encourage take-up of smoking by young people. Visual media, despite restrictions, reinforce or at least fail to challenge the cultural position of smoking. There is research evidence at the group and societal level that starting to smoke regularly is an act of conformity rather than rebellion. The cultural position of reckless driving is different. Apart from motor sport, traditional car chase films usually have associations with criminal activity, and this is still evident in film and video games. The image of a reckless speeder is a lone, male outlaw. This is not a socially integrative icon.

It would seem that there is a disproportionately inadequate response by society and the governments they elect to the manufacture and marketing of tobacco products. This is both a national and global issue, as restrictions imposed in the developed world, where tobacco companies are based, are ignored elsewhere. The regulation of the international tobacco industry appears to be a half-hearted approach at best given its record at marketing such a drug to young people. Elsewhere one can see much greater restrictions on other drugs such as cannabis, or even hard drugs such as cocaine and heroin, aimed at protecting young people. When first introduced to England, seventeenth-century anti-smoking campaigner, King James I imposed 4000 per cent duty upon tobacco. This may be more appropriate given the relative damage caused by the drug, but this would be socially unacceptable. The cultural embeddedness of smoking, even in a society fully informed of the dangers of its use, inhibits us from properly evaluating the risk associated with it.

8 Risk Communication and the Media
by Shulamit Ramon

This chapter[1] will focus on the role of the media in communicating risk within the context of mental ill health. I will be arguing that the media has an important role to play in this context, because of the highly uncertain, ambiguous and ambivalent meaning attached to mental ill health globally, but especially in post-modern societies. How it carries out this role, the issues encountered in this process and the messages given by the media will be looked at too, in the context of Australia, Italy and the UK.

The role the media occupies in communicating risk is multiple, as it engages in:

* reflecting the views of others;
* responding to these views;
* shaping public opinion.

All of these tasks require interaction with other opinion formers, making decisions about the credibility of sources of information, making decisions about the specific slant given to information, what to emphasise in the reflective responses received, and in which direction to re-shape the on-going debate or the final contribution. Thus, the media acts also in a censorship, editorial and leadership capacity.

The recipient of a specific media communication has the choice of accepting it, rejecting it, agreeing in part, switching off both literally and mentally, and choosing an altogether other media vehicle. Yet, under certain conditions, the choice is more limited than this list of options implies.

The limiting conditions pertain to what makes us dependent in the first place on the media as a major channel of communication. Presently we depend on the media to provide us with:

* information/knowledge;
* entertainment, or taking our minds off our concerns, small or big;
* help in decision-making, that is, to make our minds up when we are unclear as to what our position on an issue is, or whose opinion to trust.

---

1   This chapter was written during my sabbatical at the Institute for Advanced Studies at LaTrobe University, Melbourne, Australia. I would like to use this opportunity to thank the institute for the support given to me there.

These objectives are not mutually exclusive as, for example, entertainment can include information and can help us in making decisions through its emotional appeal no less than through the information conveyed.

The evidence is that we globally depend more and more on the media and from an earlier age.

The relatively new and growing global dependence on electronic means of communication raises the interesting issue as to whether Internet sites constitute media or scientific arenas. In so far as all Internet sites are controlled by their creators as to the direction the site will take and who has the right to respond/raise issues, they exercise editorial and leadership roles, not unlike the media, some with focus on entertainment while others focus on either more scientific information or on a shared issue of concern.

The existence of the Internet is clearly enabling a more global communication to take place and virtual communities of shared interest to be created. In the field of mental illness this enables users, carers and professionals to each choose with whom to communicate and at what level to do so.

During the last year I have been a passive member of a user-led regional website, which for most of the time consists of four people communicating with each other a couple of times per day, covering a range of topics from trivial everyday detail to their feelings about being categorised as mentally ill, including experiences and views they have of policy options. Occasionally someone else responds either with a reference to another source of information (usually an Internet site), or with a critical comment on an issue discussed by the core group. The sense is that the core group has indeed created a bond of trust, and even when its members disagree with each other, they have reached the level at which this can be expressed and allowed to pass. The trust thus created would make them believe more readily in communication about risk coming from one of them than from the outside. Issues of risk have already been aired on the site in the form of debates about the usefulness of medication versus its side effects, treatment within psychiatric wards and secure units, their ability to take risks in terms of engaging in non-illness activities and their insistence of being both ill and able – mentally and socially – at the same time.

Why are they happy with all of this to be shared by many others whom they do not know? Obviously the use of the Internet is cheaper than phone calls, video or teleconferences, but is sharing what feels often as intimate information worth the lower economic cost? Or perhaps sharing is one of the aims of the exercise and satisfaction is generated from knowing that others are influenced by their experiences?

If I were to divulge information they gave on the site, or use it for research purposes, I would have needed to secure some form of ethical permission first, even though the number of people with access to the site is unlimited.

A PhD student of mine, who is also a service user, was refused permission to use the content of a website of a network of which she is a member because of her mental ill health, on grounds that the membership has not been consulted. She was allowed though to send a questionnaire to all members of the site; but had a very low rate of response from the membership. This episode highlights the editorial capacity of those running a website, and the fine line between exercising ethical considerations and censorship, an issue of importance within the context of communicating risk in any health field.

Complexity, ambiguity and ambivalence in mental illness and mental health communication

The heading of mental illness covers an extensive range of behaviours, beliefs, thoughts and emotions, so vast that it does not constitute a continuum any longer. If we add to it mental health – defined not only as the absence of mental ill health but as encompassing mental well-being – the complexity entailed is even greater, likely to be all the more confusing. The complexity implies that identifying risk, communicating risk, and decision-making with regard to risk, are rendered complex, if not unmanageable, tasks.

The complexity is not simply a function of the vastness, but also of the need to interpret such phenomena within the context of an individual and their social environment as to its meaning, as only rarely would there be a clear-cut understanding by an outsider of the situation and often by the individual themself exhibiting signs of potential mental ill health.

Diagnostic systems have been put in place in the attempt to make both sense and order of this complexity, as well as to enable professionals to reach decisions as to the most suitable interventions. Part of the assessment process undertaken by professionals, credited with a social mandate to do so, is to assess risk, make predictions of potential risk and reach decisions as to how to manage it.

At present the American and European diagnostic manuals for mental ill health cite some four hundred categories. These cover a huge range of behaviours, beliefs, emotions, thoughts, and not less wide a range of symptoms (containing risk indicators) and prognostic predictions (or risk predictors) as to the likelihood of people to whom those diagnostic labels are attached will recover in full, partially, or not recover at all from the negative health impact of the assumed illness.

Furthermore, the range covers categories defined as distress, some defined as disturbance, and still others as illness, and disease. These distinctions also convey an assumed sliding degree of risk each brings with it.

It is also a sobering thought to know that in the history of these manuals only one category has ever been removed from it, that of homosexuality. In the 1980s the editors/authors concluded that there is insufficient evidence to identify this behaviour as a mental distress/disturbance/illness/disease, after more than a hundred years in which the opposite was claimed with equal impunity. The evidence for and against perceiving homosexuality as a mental illness category has not changed overnight or over the years. It is only the interpretation of homosexuality by psychiatrists which has changed, as the latter lived through the experience of gay people emerging from the shadows, refusing to be treated as abnormal even if their sexual orientation differs from that of the majority, and taking a collective action to ensure their citizenship rights.

Some categories have changed names – such as from moral insanity (in the nineteenth century) to psychopathy (in the early twentieth century) and to inadequate personality (in the 1970s), currently becoming known as personality disorder (as renamed in the 1990s) with ten subcategories, one of which is titled 'unspecified personality disorder'. There is no evidence to suggest the behaviour of people thus labelled has changed, or that the assumed underlying causes for it differ now, thus begging the question of what has led to changing the label. In this case it would seem that the unease felt by psychiatrists themselves of labelling people with ordinary levels of intellectual intelligence exhibiting varied symptoms of mental ill health which do not form a known cluster (syndrome), coupled with largely socially undesirable behaviours, has led them to experiment with changing old for new labels which seem more meaningful within the specific historical context. The intermittent admission by many psychiatrists of not knowing of effective interventions for these people helped to sustain the experiment, even though they continued to be required to act as social control agents for this group by formal law and order enforcers, such as the UK Home Office.

The unending increase in the number of diagnostic categories and subcategories can be seen as an attempt to refine our knowledge, but also as an attempt to retain control of what has become unwieldy, uncertain and doubtful knowledge.

The critique of this diagnostic approach from within the mental health system has likewise been ongoing, gaining momentum at certain times, and linked to socio-cultural changes in our generic understanding of life rather than of mental health or mental ill health as such. Until the second half of the twentieth century most of the critique came from psychologists, psychiatrists and social workers. It was based on finding logical flaws in the system, internal contradictions between its assumed value base (benevolence and respect of patients) and the actual values adhered to in practice (over-emphasis on social control), at times disagreeing with its underlying philosophical and scientific base (for example the value of subjective, individualised experience, and the inadequacy of positivistic methodology to the study of mental health). Yet the more powerful critique came from sociologists, who were outsiders to the system. Goffman (1961), Scheff (1975; 1999) and Garfinkel (1965) exposed the internal logic of the psychiatric diagnostic system as one in which the significance attached to signs of risk would usually exaggerate the potential risk implied, making psychiatrists usually recommend treatment options which assumed the worst possible scenario in terms of risk to others and to the person themself, and hence to adopting the least respectful option in terms of preserving the person's civil rights. This critique was made all the more influential because Goffman and Garfinkel in particular used emotionally powerful metaphors to describe the impact of the system. The metaphors include 'Total Institutions' (to describe psychiatric hospitals, prisons and army barracks); 'The Moral Career of the Mentally Ill Patient' (to describe the internal identification of oneself as mentally ill forever, after being incarcerated and described by others as morally deficient); and 'Degradation Ceremonies' (Garfinkel 1965) (describing how the past is being re-interpreted once someone is depicted as mentally ill). These sociologists, followed by protagonists of what has become known as 'anti-psychiatry' in the late 1960s and the 1970s (Laing 1967), were denouncing the use of psychiatry for the far-reaching consequences of labelling of people on the basis of rather flimsy evidence. These consequences were usually justified on the basis of projecting avoidable risk to the public and to the person.

The critique of the diagnostic manuals continues, demonstrating convincingly considerable holes in this knowledge base (Boyle 2002; Bentall 2004), and therefore doubting the logic of decisions related to risk assessment. Yet the application of the diagnostic manual continues too, largely unabashed and unimpacted by the critique.

The projected negative risk implied by the application of the manuals is in fact multidimensional, constituting potentially the following types:

1   deterioration in everyday functioning;
2   increase in unhappiness, despair and loss of self confidence;
3   reduced ability to make rational decisions and to distinguish between the real and the unreal;
4   potential harm to self;
5   potential harm to others;
6   loss of social status;

7   loss of liberty and civic rights;
8   loss of autonomy, self-agency and control over one's life;
9   loss of intimate and peer group relationships;
10   loss of ambitions;
11   loss of earnings;
12   living with long-term stigma;
13   living with long-term poverty;
14   living permanently with medication and its side-effects.

Statistically the probability of these risks materialising when mentally ill are very small with the categories from which many people suffer, such as anxiety and depression. Although making people very unhappy, at times desperate and unable to function normally, most people recover within a relatively short time and the recovery is in full, even though they become more vulnerable in the sense of a greater likelihood for depression to reoccur than in people who have never had it.

For the tiny minority suffering from psychosis, (the seven in a thousand) most of the risks listed above are real. Yet for them too, longitudinal research has demonstrated that 50–68 per cent recover in full (Ciompi 1980; Harding et al. 1987; Harrison et al. 2001). Such a recovery is more likely to happen to people in Western societies with continued family support, with higher education and in good physical health. People in the poor Third World have, however, demonstrated consistently higher and quicker rates of recovery than in the First World, largely due to experiencing much less stigma and to being less cut off socially (Warner 1985; 1994).

For a long time these known positive outcomes were kept under wraps within professional circles, giving the public the message of unavoidable chronicity and no hope for people with psychosis. It is only in the last ten years that these findings have gained part of the attention they deserve, mainly due to the efforts of articulate service users who have adopted the concept of recovery from mental illness in a new meaning which focuses on regaining control over one's life, rather than either getting rid of symptoms or going back to previous, normal functioning (Deegan 1996; Roberts and Wolfson 2004). The recovery studies highlight the importance of the context in which the person lives in terms of likely genuine support they may be receiving and giving themselves, as well as in terms of socio-economic characteristics, such as education.

Moreover, the recovery process – that is, the period in which people get out of their illness and begin to live outside it (Davidson 2003) – literally requires that they will be *taking risks* in terms of expanding their control over their own lives, of overcoming the isolation they went into during the time they struggled with their mental illness, of beginning to give to others rather than be takers, of trusting themselves anew and re-trusting others as well. All of these require a high level of risk for someone who is fragile to put to one side the components which have become their known reality for the sake of what has become to an extent an unknown reality, even if experienced before. The possibility of recovery cannot be entertained without risk-taking being shared by the person who has been ill, by their informal and formal carers as well (Roberts and Wolfson 2004; Rapaport 2005).

Risk in mental illness and in mental health entails always both risk avoidance side by side with risk-taking, inevitably creating complex interlinked components and processes (Ramon 2005).

Patricia Deegan is a well-known protagonist of the users' recovery perspective; she is both a service user and a psychologist. In 1996 she stated, 'Professionals must embrace the concept of the dignity of risk, and the right to failure if they are to be supportive of us' (Deegan 1996, 97). Thus, in communicating risk in mental illness and health, the media would need to reflect both risk avoidance and risk-taking.

If the media is to reflect adequately on current mental health issues, it would need to take into account the diversity of views as to the aetiology of mental ill health, not less than that of symptomatology already mentioned above. Recovery provides one recent example of the diversity of the professional discourse itself, to the point that it is difficult to talk about one such discourse.

Those who share a medical perspective tend to believe in the supremacy of not only the biological/bio-chemical origin of mental illness but also in that of a clinical approach to mental ill health and mental health.

Those adhering to a social perspective tend to accept not only the limitations of a biochemical approach, but also of the clinical approach to service users and their families, as well as the actual harm that such approaches lead to by ignoring the social, which includes the impact of social structures, culture, economy and politics on the development and maintaining of both mental illness and health.

The psychological perspective also does not constitute one perspective, but a number of approaches ranging from the most behavioural to the most psychoanalytic.

In some approaches the social and the psychological come together (Ramon and Williams 2005); it is rare however to find an approach which has managed to put together the medical, the social and the psychological in a coherent framework which does justice to the different emphasis each brings (Double 2005). This spills over from conceptual models to practice, and to different views about the appropriateness of prevalent research methods.

Thus the domain of mental illness and health is indeed contested. Moreover, in a moment of truth, the lack of sufficient knowledge is acknowledged (see below the quotation from Dr Pemberton in the *Daily Telegraph* of 16 March 2005).

The three countries from which examples are given in this text are similar in undergoing considerable change in their psychiatric system in the last 25 years. All three have moved from a system in which psychiatric hospitals constituted the core service, to one in which very few such institutions are left, being replaced by a mixture of psychiatric wards in general hospitals, community mental health teams, specialists teams in Australia and the UK for crisis and/or early intervention, working with people in need of long-term support, a lot more attention to education and employment, more psycho-educational work with users and their families, and much more articulate user voice (Ramon 2000; Repper and Perkins 2003; Healy and Renouf 2005).

Italy differs in having more generic community mental health teams, some of them with beds, a more informal relationship among the different disciplines and between patients and professionals, and in particular a transformative de-institutionalisation process which has also impacted on the general population (Mosher and Burti 1989; Ramon 1990; Mezzina 2005).

It would be fair to state that the rapid changes in the three systems have not necessarily been internalised by many of the professionals working in these systems, and certainly not by the general public, including the media.

Perhaps unsurprisingly, these radical changes have been perceived as controversial in each of these three countries, but to different degrees. In the UK, a government minister claimed in 1997 that community care has failed, even though existing evidence does not support this claim (Leff 1997). In Australia, recent claims have been made that early discharge and an insufficient number of beds in hospitals led to an increase in suicide by a small group of people around five weeks after the discharge (*The Age*, 24 July 2005, p. 6). However, the article also includes a leading advocate's claim of abuse by staff in these admission wards, and the story of one patient who complained of such an incidence of physical abuse. Similar claims are not made in Italy, even though in many ways its psychiatric reform has been the more radical of the three countries; considerable regional and local disparities in service provision are known to exist (Ramon and Savio 2000).

Challenge that mental illness and health poses for the media

The analysis provided above has highlighted that the media does not have a straightforward job in reflecting, shaping and responding in the context of mental health and illness. The complexity, and even more so the ambiguity, described challenges the media to dispense with any simplistic presentation. However, the pull of over-simplification may be equally strong, as many media people believe that the public cannot tolerate a high degree of complexity, and that the media itself is the message (Philo 1996). Speaking about the depiction of youth in the media, Hartley (1992) proposed that whenever presented with a 'dirt category' (that is, a category which contains a high level of ambiguity and ambivalence) the media is tempted to opt for simplistic messages because they reduce the uncertainty generated by ambiguity, and convey a false sense of safety for the readers/viewers. Faced with a contested background, considerable degree of change and of competing approaches and stakeholders, the media itself will be more influenced by the socio-political stance of the specific medium, as presented either by the editors or/and the owners, than when presented with a more black and white context.

Specifically pertaining to risk, the 'liquid' not easily definable quality of risk in mental health – to borrow Bauman's (2003) use of the concept with respect to modern types of relationships – may therefore mean that most media would opt for over-simplification. In the post 9/11 times in which we live any negative risk is magnified and treated as an immediate threat, and the suspension of human rights and civil liberties is more easily and quickly applied (Bauman 2002).

Media reflection, shaping and responding in the context of mental health and illness: form and content

We will turn now to look at *how* the media carries out the role and tasks outlined above, and the *content* it communicates.

The how is partly dependent on the specific type of media: newspapers emphasise the written language, while TV, films and videos provide a multimedia coverage. Yet the how contains many more possibilities with each specific media type.

Newspapers can play with the amount of space and location of the item (for example front page, back page), the use of headline, the type of emphasis on emotional versus intellectual or factual coverage, attributing the information to others and selecting who to attribute it to. It can decide whether to criticise the particular version or not, to trivialise, demonise or glorify a particular piece of information.

The story of Cornelia Rau, an Australian citizen who absconded from a psychiatric hospital and was then interned by the Australian authorities as an illegal immigrant for a year made many headlines in the newspapers in Australia in July 2005. Some opted to have her story on the front page, though it was a story not told by her; some to have her sister's story on the front page (the sister is a journalist); and some to have coverage only of the official report of the inquiry which followed her identification by her parents from a photo displayed in a newspaper. All newspapers had also a picture of Ms Rau, but differed in where they displayed it and its size.

Multimedia types of communication have at their disposal all of the above, plus the use of images, colour, shade, voice, and a more comprehensive storytelling medium.

Australian TV channels differed in opting to interview Ms Rau's parents, her sister, her lawyer and/or the civil servant who wrote the inquiry report, as Ms Rau herself could not be interviewed because she was back in a psychiatric hospital. Both newspapers and all TV channels reported in full the formal apology given by the Australian Prime Minister to Ms Rau about the way she was treated by the immigration authorities.

Photos of Ms Rau and other prominent people in this case appeared in colour in both newspapers and the TV. However, in the article of 24 July the photos are almost all in black, reinforcing the message of doom and gloom which the content stressed.

The big and most sensational headline in the UK in March 2005 was a case in which a black man who was a voluntary patient in an inner city psychiatric ward in a general hospital killed and ate part of the body of a man who was his friend. The case was further complicated by the fact that the killer was put in a cell with another patient in a specially secure hospital and had murdered the other patient/prisoner, after being sentenced to life detention in that psychiatric hospital.

All of the tabloids put his picture on the front page in such a way that even without the gory caption one could sense a very unsavoury person/story from it. None of the quality papers put that photo in, despite differences in their coverage of the case.

In this case both TV and the newspapers interviewed professionals and the managers of the specific mental health trust, and some of the relatives of another recent killing by a patient in the mental health system. It is unclear why none of the relatives of the victim in this specific case were interviewed, or whether they were approached and refused to be interviewed. This is an example how by an unexplained omission a story gets a particular slant.

And just in case the reader is perplexed about the likelihood of being killed in the UK by a person known to its mental health services, let me outline the facts: the UK has about 40 cases of such killings per year, compared to an overall number of 600 killings, 560 of which are committed by people judged to be sane. The figures have not increased in the wake of hospital closure; if any, they have come slightly down, as demonstrated effectively in a study carried out by two eminent forensic psychiatrists (Taylor and Gunn 1999). Indeed, in one paper covering the infamous killing mentioned above there is an article on the same page by the mother of a murdered teenager shot dead by another young man, apparently without a motive (*Daily Telegraph*, 16 March 2005, p. 4). The mother mentions that there are 260 killings per year in the UK of this nature, yet only in exceptional circumstances do such killings get the coverage the one carried out by a mentally ill person did in terms of space and prominence. It would seem that the significance the media is attaching to different types of killings is not closely related to the number of people thus dying, but to the salacious, or unusual, way in which they were killed.

In contrast, mental health news which got to prominence in Italy was one in which it was discovered that local hospital workers in a southern city were siphoning considerable sums earmarked for the hospital to their own pockets (*Maurizio Constanzo Show*, Canale 5, 1985).

The whistleblowers were other employees in the same hospital, who took a courageous stance in an area known for its Mafia grasp. The opposition MP to whom the details were given opted to create a political scandal, but also to organise a concert with nationally well-known artists for the patients within the grounds of the hospital. Newspapers and TV coverage focused on the poor physical state of the hospital on the one hand, and on the concert with the patients on the other. The *Maurizio Constanzo Show* combines a mixture of items every evening, ranging from the appearance of lightly clad starlets to that of priests – titillating and serious issues put together. The decision to put this item within the context of the programme reflects on its significance as a human-angle story with a gossip perspective about the joint involvement of well-known artists and politicians.

Pertaining to the *content*, even in the description of the forms the media has selected outlined above it was difficult to fully distinguish form from content, as the two seem to be used to reinforce the central message the medium wants to portray.

All of the examples given thus far contain clear messages related to *risk*, albeit of a diverse nature.

In the case of Cornelia Rau the risk is to the person-patient from a state system aimed at improving the safety and prosperity of Australian citizens, namely the immigration authorities. The catalogue of misunderstandings, stereotyping because of colour and level of articulation, the deep disrespect for most basic civic rights, the treatment of potentially illegal immigrants as dangerous criminals, and the ignorance regarding serious mental ill health is unending. Although Ms Rau seems to have been at times out of most basic self control and socially acceptable behaviour, therefore perhaps at risk to herself first and foremost, the immigration officers were preoccupied with attempting to secure her deportation to Germany rather than with her state of health. The Australian media seems to have had a field day in describing all of the above most of the time, and only at the end of the coverage of the affair do they raise the obvious concerns of having a service funded by the tax payer which is devoid of both professionalism and ethical considerations. Although Ms Rau is described as being seriously mentally ill it is not suggested at any stage that she presented a risk to others.

Likewise in the article on suicide the risk focused upon is to oneself, with the mental health system being accused of misjudging when patients should be discharged and at times of allowing abuse to take place. However, the main responsibility is put at the door of the federal and state governments which fund the service at an insufficient level according to the different media.

In the British case the risk identified was clearly to others and of a very severe nature. The professionals were accused of misdiagnosis on a big scale, especially as it transpired that they had reached the decision to free the patient from hospital detention against the advice of the Home Office. The patient was known to have been violent in the past, which usually is treated as a predictor for the future and raises alarm bells. Psychiatrists and a social worker were signalled out as the people who made this gross misjudgement more than once over a period of a few weeks prior to the killing. The views of these professionals were not canvassed; most likely they could not give interviews for judicial reasons. However, the media presented the view of the representative of the health trust in which they worked, who justified the decision on the basis of what was known at the time, namely that the patient was ready to come to the psychiatric ward of his own volition, that he took more responsibility for looking after himself and they were sure that he was taking the medication as he did not demonstrate psychotic symptoms.

While most of the media were happy to highlight the flaws in the judgement of these professionals and to see them as guilty of not locking up this patient and thus prevent him from carrying out the brutal killing, one newspaper asked a psychiatrist who often writes for the newspaper for his view. Headed 'No one can ever say for sure whether a patient poses a risk', Dr Pemberton went on to say:

> Risk is not an easy thing to assess. For psychiatrists, it forms the major part of their job, but it is also one of the most difficult parts. As the case of Peter Bryan shows, sometimes they don't get it right ... There was nothing in his behaviour to indicate the horrific crime he was about to commit. This is the unfortunate truth about psychiatry: psychiatrists trained in diagnosing mental illness, are not, contrary to popular opinion, able to read people's minds ... Psychiatrists will never be able to say for sure whether a patient poses a risk. All they can do is assess each case to the best of their abilities. (Daily Telegraph, 16 March 2005, p. 4 – The Daily Telegraph is a politically right-of-centre newspaper)

This apologetic statement for the state of our scientific knowledge was not what most of the media wanted to hear in this particular case, where they clearly wanted to somehow reassure the public – and themselves – that there *must* be certainty in this type of risk assessment.

Another quality newspaper went even further than the *Daily Telegraph* in using the occasion to point out that the UK is admitting too many people with mental ill health to its psychiatric wards, and that instead it should develop resources in the community which will enable people to be treated as early as possible, when the likely risk is much easier to treat and to contain (Riddle, *Observer*, 20 March 2005 p. 28). The *Observer* is a politically left-of-centre newspaper.

To judge by the fury of the other papers, the *Observer* was making a very courageous stand, as all other newspapers were clamouring to demand that more people will be admitted on a compulsory basis for an indefinite period as a way of tackling this potential risk. For example, the *Daily Mirror* (despite being left-of-centre politically) opts to describe in considerable details the letter the killer–patient has sent to the father of a much earlier victim (who was not eaten), titled 'Hannibal Letter', alluding to the film *Hannibal Lector* about a killer who ate his victims (*Daily Mirror*, 16 March 2005, p. 5). It would seem that the differences in being a tabloid or a quality newspaper is more significant to the coverage of mental illness than the political orientation of a newspaper.

The risk issue in the Italian example is focused on actual physical harm to patients by a group which exploited its professional status for personal illegal gains at the expense of highly vulnerable people who could not defend themselves against this exploitation. The story also demonstrated that not everyone working for the system shares this greed and readiness to exploit, reflected by the act of the whistleblowers.

Moreover, the influential people outside the system were ready to both blow up the case and offer solidarity to the patients–victims in addition to making sure that the exploitation will be stopped, that the basic physical conditions would be improved and that the exploiters will be duly punished.

In a way it is easier to focus on a clear physical neglect and risk issue than on a more psycho-social one, as the meaning is unambiguous.

The media does not raise the issue of what may happen to the whistleblowers and to the patients once the halo of this event disappears, reflecting on the short-fuse nature of most media coverage.

Conclusions

The coverage in these examples highlights *how* the media communicates risks as well as *what* it does communicate in the case of mental illness. In attempting to respond to the challenge of reflecting, shaping and responding to issues of mental ill health, the media usually opts for an over-simplification of the issues at stake. This reduces the level of ambiguity involved while increasing the assumed degree of certainty in the information provided. Thus, in Mary Douglas's terms, danger is responded to and controlled; purity is maintained by homing in on only one or two elements at most (Douglas 1966). The fact that the reality of mental ill health for users, carers or professionals often does not correspond to this new painting/ interpretation of it does not matter much, because the media speaks mostly to the uninformed who wish to be reassured about their understanding of mental ill health and indeed it offers them such a reassurance. The specific interpretations given by different types of media differ in part in accordance with the overall political ideology a medium adheres to, but especially in which population groups it seeks to reach. Thus, quality newspapers reflect and enable greater complexity to come across in their interpretation of the risk component than tabloids do, even if in so doing they cross the party political line they usually follow. Another safeguard against over-simplification, in evidence in Italian media coverage (Kemali et al. 1989), takes place when the general population is ready to accept the complexity of mental ill health. Following the attempts of the reformers of the mental health system there to engage the general public in events related to the reform and in a better understanding of mental ill health, the media too was able to portray the issues entailed in a less simplistic way than was the case for the British media at the same period (Ramon and Savio 2000).

Risk communication is a sensitive issue for all media, especially in this day and age. Risk in an uncertain and liquid field such as mental illness is even more so, but the sensitivity does not necessarily imply readiness to look for an in-depth understanding and interpretation, as the latter would of necessity call for multi-perspectives to be produced and muddy the water.

The fear of risk also implies an overwhelming focus on risk avoidance, with little interest demonstrated in risk-taking, even though the media is focusing on risk-taking in sport, business, entertainment and politics all the time. Thus, positive developments in mental health are hardly ever covered because they all contain a high degree of risk-taking. It is only in reflecting on mental illness through artistic achievements – such as poetry, novels, films, painting – that the media allows itself at times to recognise the insight which mental ill health offers to humanity.

9 Social Life of Risk Communication
by Dawn Hillier

The power of symbolic systems to mediate and organise people's experience of the world is central to contemporary cultures. Multiple factors dynamically converge to support children's and adults' progress in complex symbol systems. There has been an expansion over the past 20 years on narrative concerning risk literacy development that strives to capture the embeddedness of people's learning and understanding of health risk in meaningful, socially rich, scaffolding exchanges with more knowledgeable others.

Once upon a time... Risk messages contained within stories and fairy tales

With these few words we are transported to a different realm, filled with magic and wonder and untold possibilities. As little children we were enchanted by the adventures of beautiful princesses surrounded by fairy godmothers, wicked old witches, nasty stepmothers and evil queens. We carry these and the dreams of triumph of good over evil and happily-ever-afters into our worlds as adults.

Often embedded in fairy tales are significant cultural symbols about how we should live our lives, what is right and wrong and what dangers lie ahead of us. Risk is communicated in both direct and indirect ways; for example, while sitting with a three-year-old visitor watching the 1993 cartoon film *Snow White in Happily Ever After*, I became aware of a number of health risk message embedded in the script. The first was portrayed by the owl character that smoked smelly cigars, coughed constantly and had trouble breathing and smelling. The owl's health risk from smoking became a secondary one to the absolute risk of dying as a result of being suspended above a caldron of boiling water, held only by a burning rope. The owl has a coughing episode and his sidekick played by a bat, tells him, 'You've gotta quit smoking boss – it'll kill you,' generating the response, 'I'm about to be owl stew and he's worried about smoking.' At the conclusion of the film another character took the cigar from the owl's mouth and suddenly he could take a deep breathe saying, 'I can smell again'. Bat replied, 'With your cigar you always smelled.'

Fairy tales and children's stories often simplistically relay positive messages to children. Fairy-tale symbolism resonates with most of us but the films typically have a very American message: good will triumph. And what is more, many books, movies, commercials and television shows are essentially retellings of fairy-tale themes.

Fairy tales reflect the conditions, ideas, tastes and values of the societies in which they were created. Due to their symbolism, it is quite often very difficult to see how remarkably they comment on reality. It has been demonstrated by psychologists and educators time and again that stories and fairy tales do influence the manner in which children conceive the world and their places in it even before they begin to read (Zipes 1986, xii).

In contrast to the conventional approach which views communications as the sending of a message from a communicator to a recipient, storytelling is based on a more interactive view of communication. Because the listener imaginatively recreates the story in their own mind, the story is not perceived as coming from outside, but rather as something that is part of the listener's own identity. The idea becomes the listener's own.

When used effectively, storytelling offers numerous advantages over more traditional communication techniques.

- Stories communicate ideas holistically, conveying a rich yet clear message, and so they are an excellent way of communicating complicated ideas and concepts in an easy-to-understand form. Stories therefore allow people to convey tacit knowledge that might otherwise be difficult to articulate; in addition, because stories are told with feeling, they can allow people to communicate more than they realise they know.

- Storytelling provides the context in which knowledge arises as well as the knowledge itself, and hence can increase the likelihood of accurate and meaningful knowledge transfer.

- Stories are an excellent vehicle for learning, as true learning requires interest, which abstract principles and impersonal procedures rarely provide.

- Stories are memorable – their messages tend to stick and they get passed on.

- Stories can provide a living, breathing example of how to do something and why it works rather than telling people what to do, hence people are more open to their lessons.

- Stories therefore often lead to direct action – they can help to close the knowing–doing gap (the difference between knowing how to do something and actually doing it).

- Storytelling can help to make communication more human – not only do they use natural day-to-day language, but they also elicit an emotional response as well as thoughts and actions.

- Stories can nurture a sense of community and help to build relationships.

- People enjoy sharing stories – stories enliven and entertain.

A simple story can communicate a complex multi-dimensioned idea, not simply by transmitting information as a message, but by actively involving the listeners in co-creating that idea. Furthermore, as a story is told and retold, it changes, and so the knowledge embodied in it is constantly being developed and built upon. This can be seen clearly in the genre known as soap opera.

Soap opera

The power of soap opera is that it is immediate and historic, claims Hobson (2003). Soap opera began as a need to attract audiences to the newly emerging medium of radio and has developed and evolved into a genre which has spread from radio to television and from America to Britain, Australia and countries across the world. It is a genre that has contributed significantly to the continued success of broadcasting. Soap opera has a core set of characters and locations and is transmitted more than three times a week for 52 weeks a year. The main focus of the narrative is on the everyday personal and emotional lives of its characters and creates the illusion that the characters and the location exist and continue to operate whether the viewers are there or not. Viewers are invited to drop in and share the characters lives, but the illusion depends on the credibility that life goes on when the viewers are not watching.

Entertainment-education strategy is based on Bandura's (1977a and 1977b) social cognitive theory, which posits that individuals learn new behaviours by observing and imitating the behaviour of others, who serve as role models. Another underlying principle is that individuals may increase their self-efficacy, or sense of their ability to carry out a task, by seeing individuals similar to themselves perform the task successfully. This makes entertainment-education a suitable approach for efforts to reduce unintended pregnancy and HIV infection, since self-efficacy is associated with contraceptive use among women at risk of these events (Galavotti et al. 1995).

In summary, exposure to characters in soap operas can lead to parasocial interaction between certain audience members and characters in the soap opera. Parasocial relationships are the seemingly face-to-face interpersonal relationships which can develop between a viewer and a mass media personality (Horton and Wohl 1956). Horton and Wohl argued that when a parasocial relationship is established, the media consumer appreciates the values and motives of the media character, often viewing them as a counsellor, comforter and model. Rubin and Perse (1987) argued that parasocial interaction consists of three audience dimensions – cognitive, affective, and behavioural.

- *Cognitively-oriented parasocial interaction* is the degree to which audience members pay careful attention to the characters in a media message and think about its educational content after their exposure (Papa et al. 2000; Sood and Rogers 2000).

- *Affectively-oriented parasocial interaction* is the degree to which an audience member identifies with a particular media character, and believes that their interests are joined (Burke 1945). The stronger the identification, the more likely that character's behaviour will affect the audience member.

- *Behaviourally-oriented parasocial interaction* is the degree to which individuals overtly react to media characters, for instance, by 'talking' to these characters, or by conversing with other audience members about them. Such conversations may influence audience members' thinking about an educational issue and motivate them to change their behaviour in a specific way.

These parasocial relationships often prompt peer conversations among viewers. Casual observation in a variety of social settings, for example, the hairdresser's, the local market, and so on, provides numerous examples of how soap operas stimulate conversations among listeners, creating a social learning environment for social change. Audience members can share their similar and different perceptions of the information presented in the programme. They may talk about considering or adopting socially desirable behaviours that are highlighted in the programme. These interpersonal discussions create a social learning environment in which people learn from one another. Collective efficacies emerge when people share ideas about the health risks facing their community and discuss ways of confronting resistance to their plans for change.

Example from radio soap opera in St Lucia

In 1990, St Lucia's population was about 136000 and it grew by about 1.2 per cent per year to 2000 (Registrar of Civil Status and Statistics Department 1994; Population Reference Bureau (PRB) 2000). The total fertility rate of 3.8 lifetime births per woman in 1980 declined to 2.6 by 1997 (Statistics Department 1994; PRB 1997). The contraceptive prevalence rate remained roughly constant at about 55 per cent from 1988 to 1997 (Jagdeo 1990; PRB 1997). Around 62 per cent of pregnancies were unintended in 1988 (Jagdeo 1990), and 21 per cent of births were to women younger than 20 in 1991 (Statistics Department 1994).

Catholicism is the predominant religion in St Lucia, but Seventh-Day Adventist and evangelical Protestant churches represent a growing minority. Many St Lucians choose not to marry, but instead cohabit or enter visiting unions (in which the partners do not live together); as a result, 85 per cent of births occur out of wedlock (Ebanks 1985). This is similar to arrangements in some parts of Ghana (Hillier 1992).

In an endeavour to address the family planning issues, an entertainment-education radio soap opera, *Apwe Plezi*,[1] was broadcast from February 1996 to September 1998 in St Lucia. The programme promoted family planning, HIV prevention and other social development themes.

Vaughan et al. (2000) assessed the programme's effects through analyses of data from nationally representative pre-test and post-test surveys, focus-group discussions and other qualitative and quantitative sources. The results showed that among the 1238 respondents to the post-test survey, 35 per cent had listened to *Apwe Plezi*, including 12 per cent who listened at least once weekly. Multivariate analyses show significant effects of both time and listenership categories on several knowledge, attitude and behaviour variables. For example, 16 per cent of post-test respondents knew a slang term for condoms that was created for the radio programme, and the proportions of respondents who considered it acceptable for husbands to have sex partners outside their marriage declined from 27 per cent in the pre-test to 14 per cent in the post-test survey. Compared with non-listeners, regular listeners were more likely to trust family planning workers (83 per cent versus 72 per cent) and considered a significantly lower number of children the ideal (2.5 versus 2.9). Fourteen per cent of listeners reported having adopted a family planning method as a result of listening to the programme.

Vaughan et al. (2000) concluded that *Apwe Plezi* influenced listeners to increase their awareness of contraceptives, improve important attitudes about fidelity and family relations, and adopt family planning methods. Important lessons for entertainment-education programmers include that programme reach, and therefore effects, can be limited by competition with other programming, and that monitoring listeners' perceptions is essential to detect and correct misinterpretations of programme messages.

---

1   The name Apwe Plezi derives from the Creole proverb 'Apwe plezi c'est la pain', or 'After the pleasure comes the pain' (Regis and Butler 1997).

The characters in soap operas are the key to why audiences watch the programmes. As Hobson (2003, 105) states, the chemistry of a soap opera and its audiences is one which involves a considerable commitment on the part of the viewers. The characters are so well known by the viewers but that does not mean they cannot change. But if the character does change, it has to be in a way that is appropriate and within the realistic parameters of how that character would behave. Characters must be predictable but also capable of surprise. Moreover, they must be capable of change, vulnerable but also show their depths and strengths when needed. It is they who have to cope with the vicissitudes of life. They who link the realism of the drama with the reality of everyday life; their stories are our stories and what happens in their lives must have a resonance in our lives. Moreover, characters convey the spirit of the times; for example, Baby Boomers, characterised by their legacy of commitment, feminism and environmentalism, living in a time of plenty, who cashed in the job opportunities; and Generation X, a disenfranchised generation overshadowed by the Boomers (see Coupland 1991), ranging from the young, individualistic, egocentric, hedonistic, ambitious, materialistic, market oriented, conservative and cynical, to those who see economic opportunities vanishing, youth unemployment or more importantly underemployment. It is the final group that return home to live with their parents and defer their dreams of a lifestyle that includes home ownership, marriage and children. Generation Xers have less idealism, which is seen as a luxury, and their issues are not ones of intrinsic values, they cannot afford to ask these questions – they have to pay the bills, especially as the Boomers are getting older and it is the Generation Xers who will have to support them.

The concept of good characters and bad characters seems to be redundant in relation to soap operas. As in real life, people are more complex than merely being good or bad, hero or villain (Hobson 2003, 106). Characters are multifaceted and we see their different characteristics and their intentions and behaviours with a number of other characters which allows us to judge their behaviour and understand their motivation. Accepting different characters and an understanding of their psychological complexities is possible because the nature of this genre enables the production to develop and reveal many aspects of major characters.

The cultural significance of soap operas is greater than the drama itself, because they integrate with all aspects of our lives. They become part of the narrative of our lives and they are part of our memories and the memories of our shared relationships.

What is interesting and important in the global village is that we are sharing these narratives.

Case example: communicating health messages – Hispanic experience

According to the Center for Disease Control, Hispanic people in the United States experience a disproportionate burden of preventable disease, death, and disability compared to non-minorities. Since they often have limited access to healthcare, Spanish-language telenovelas (soap operas) can serve a critical health education service when they provide accurate, timely information about health issues. By the year 2035, there will be 75 million Hispanics comprising 20 per cent of the US population. Beck et al. (2003) assert that over the past five years, Hispanic-American television households have grown by 19 per cent compared with 29 per cent growth of Spanish-dominant television households – from 3.5 million to 4.6 million.

Analysis of the 2002 Porter Novelli HealthStyles database was conducted by the Centers for Disease Control and Prevention (CDC) and Hollywood, Health & Society at the USC Annenberg Norman Lear Center. The dataset consists of responses from 21 items that were included in the national HealthStyles Survey to describe the characteristics of telenovela viewers, impact of health content in telenovelas and top sources for health information among telenovela viewers. The key findings are outlined below:

- Five percent of all respondents (n = 216) are *telenovela viewers*, that is, viewers who watch telenovelas at least a few times a month (27 per cent of Hispanics, 6 per cent of Blacks and 2 per cent of Whites).

- Hispanic, lower-income, lower-educated, and younger-age groups report more often learning something new about a health topic, taking action, making a health care choice, and providing health information to friends, family or others after hearing about a health topic on a telenovela.

- Forty-two percent of respondents rate Spanish-language TV as a top source of learning about health, behind TV news/news magazine shows (48 per cent) and health care providers (44 per cent).

- Prime time TV entertainment shows are cited as a top source of learning about health by one in three *telenovela viewers*.

- Two percent of all respondents (n=84) report they are *regular viewers*, that is, they watch telenovelas at least twice a week.

- Nearly nine out of ten (88 per cent) report knowing other friends or acquaintances who are also *regular viewers* of telenovelas.

- Four out of ten (43 per cent) *regular viewers* and 31 per cent of *all viewers* report that a telenovela storyline helped them make a health care choice.

- More than one-third (38 per cent) of Hispanics who viewed a few times a month, report that a telenovela storyline helped them make a health care choice.

- More than half (55 per cent) of *regular viewers* and 39 per cent of *all viewers* report that a telenovela storyline helped them provide important health information to their friends, family or others.

- Nearly half (48 per cent) of Hispanics who viewed a few times a month report that a telenovela storyline helped them provide important health information to their friends, family or others.

The Healthstyles findings suggest TV soap operas can serve a critical health education service by providing accurate, timely information about disease, injury and disability in their storylines for more than 38 million people who regularly watch daytime dramas. Since *regular viewers* have more health concerns and negative beliefs and practices that may contribute to poor health, and they are highly receptive to health information in the soaps, they are an important audience for accurate, easily understood health messages. When even a small percentage of viewers take action as the result of a TV soap opera, to protect or improve their own health or the health of someone they know, millions of people and their families can benefit. If soap operas fail to convey accurate information, or portray risky behaviour without the associated health consequences, there is the possibility millions of people will suffer negative effects.

Role models on television, however, often do not provide particularly helpful messages regarding health. While there are exceptions, frequent alcohol consumption, unprotected sex, poor dietary habits, cigarette smoking and using violence as a problem-solving solution are common themes.

Based on the survey findings, a list of suggestions was created for writers and producers of telenovelas; these communicators are encouraged to consider:

- topics and diseases that are most prevalent among US Hispanics (for example diabetes, homicide, HIV, prenatal care, breast/cervical cancer, vaccines for children);

- prevention information delivered or modelled by credible characters (for example checking the smoke alarm, using a seat belt, taking a daily vitamin, having regular medical check-ups, exercising);

- storylines that explore the impact of disease, injury and disability on people's lives, and how they can find help within the health care system or their local communities;

- characters with negative beliefs and poor health practices suffering the consequences (for example a smoker who is diagnosed with lung cancer or an inactive adult who finds they have diabetes);

- challenges and struggles characters face in making changes and the positive outcomes that result when they choose more positive beliefs and practices (for example the smoker who quits and stops coughing or the teen who is overweight but starts to become physically active);

- storylines with characters who have health limitations or impairment but practice healthy behaviours that contribute to their quality of life (for example an HIV-positive person who gets regular check-ups and takes their medication with care).

Television, however, cultivates an understanding of health that systematically reinforces the individual nature of disease and ignores or minimises the social, economic, and political factors that are major determinants of health. Television presents a medical, rather than a social model of health, and the medical profession is portrayed with a great deal of power and authority in the health arena. The primary methods of treating illness or diseases tend to be machines and drugs, with a heavy biomedical emphasis. Moreover, medical care, and the diseases it treats, is portrayed as apolitical and independent of larger political, economic and social concerns that are central to contemporary debates about the role of medicine in the health care system.

Social change through entertainment-education

Population Communications International (PCI), working with local partners worldwide, produces carefully researched and culturally sensitive radio and television soap operas that combine the power of storytelling with the reach of broadcast media.

Women's empowerment, health, education and safety are fundamental themes in PCI's entertainment-education programmes. The programmes address the societal factors that limit people's ability to make choices that will improve their health and educational prospects. The serial dramas are intended to motivate individuals to adopt new attitudes and behaviour by modelling behaviours that promote family health, stable communities and a sustainable environment. Each series is written, performed and produced by the creative talent in that country. From their earliest broadcast initiatives to contemporary programmes in India, Pakistan, Mexico, the United States and elsewhere in the world, improving every woman's ability to control her own destiny is central to their mission.

In the Andean Highlands, PCI's programme focuses on high maternal mortality rates, low levels of male participation in family planning and a gap between what people say they know about family planning and actual contraceptive use.

In Mexico, PCI's live radio show *Ombligos al Sol* (Bellybuttons to the Sun) engages teenagers with a mix of news, music, testimonials, expert advice, audience call-in and a mini-drama with sexual and reproductive health content.

In India and Pakistan, women continue to fight oppressive traditions epitomised by son preference, the strong social bias toward sons and adult males, which leads to sex-selective abortions and lifetime deprivation for girls and women. In Bihar, one of the northern Indian states where a PCI programme called *Taru* (launched in February 2002), fewer than two out of ten women could read and write.

Taru, the programme's 21-year-old main character, is a young woman determined to resist cultural traditions, further her education and shape a destiny outside marriage. According to the researchers (Singhal 2003) one Indian woman said she has changed after listening to the programme:

> *Earlier I used to be very rigid, but now my vision has expanded. Now I do not 'rule over' my daughters … girls can also progress. We gave so much freedom to boys while controlling the girls too much … that they shouldn't go out, shouldn't talk to people, even should not talk openly with their elder brother. Now, after listening to Taru, I have given freedom to all of them.*

Beyond the airing of such programmes, the audience will gossip about the characters and their lives, exchanging differing opinions and views of the world in which the characters live and reflect upon their own experiences in their own world.

Hot gossip: inferential risk communication

Storytelling, gossip and rumour create a mental model of the world and how the world should look, behave and respond. Gossip did not always have the negative connotations it has today. According to *Webster's Dictionary*, the word 'gossip' came from the Middle English 'godsib' or 'godsipp', meaning a godparent or sponsor. It referred to a kinship circle. Gossip at that time was more about bonding with others than today's connotation of 'idle chatter between two parties, regarding a third'.

During the last four or five decades, cultural historians, sociologists and socio-psychologists have stressed the usefulness as an approach to what the French professor in strategy and marketing Jean-Nöel Kapferer (1990) has termed 'popular reality' – the verbal culture of non-literary communities or populations and the world view it expresses. From rumours and hearsay we can sometimes gain a specific view of the fears and wishes, aggressions and presumptions of individuals and groups, whose psychology and world views are otherwise lost in generalisations.

Rumours are also increasingly used to highlight power-struggles in early modern societies and modern societies alike. Sociologists and cultural historians now see rumours not only as a tool in political or inter-elite power struggles, but also as an important mechanism in conflicts between the powerless and empowered members of a society, both as a sort of hidden resistance and critique of established society and as a disciplining mechanism on the part of the established elite in their dealings with the people.

Rumours about disease and illness draw on the rich symbolism of the body and are a way for social groups to express concerns about their relationships to the community and state. For example, the Indonesian 'AIDS Club' rumours are part of a body of contemporary legends about AIDS that have circulated globally. In their local form, however, they speak to particular concerns that urban Indonesians have about modernity and the power of the Indonesian state (cited in Butt 2005).

Social life of conversation

Chat shows are a fertile ground for communicating risk through rumour, gossip and conflict. This genre generally is concerned with creating mental noise and confusion and generating emotional responses to the issues through stress on social conformity and moral judgements. Risk messages underlie the chat show format but are inferred rather than openly stated and depend on the knowledge of risk of the audience and the participants. For example in the Sally Jessy Rafael Show, the chat show format is used to great effect as can be seen the following description of one show:

> *Scenario (shown Tuesday 18 October on ITV2 UK)*
>
> *Parents of a 15-year-old girl appeared on the show to try to persuade their daughter's 26-year-old boyfriend to leave her alone. Their objections were allegedly based on his age (and from his point of view his ethnicity). The girl already has a son by another man but spends her time with her boyfriend drinking and hanging out and not taking care of her child, neither is she going to school. Moreover, she runs away from home on a regular basis. The girl's father boasts of beating up the boyfriend for taking advantage of his daughter and accuses him of being a pimp. The visual image on screen is one of aggression and the audience gets a sense of underlying violence and mutual hostility. When the girl comes on stage her response to her father's attempt to hug her is unreceptive saying, when asked by Sally why she rejected her father's affection, that he was just putting on an act for the audience, and claiming that he does not normally show affection.*

Such stories weave people into communities or social networks of producers that constitute a kind of common sense that allows the key issues to emerge. The key message threads in this particular scenario raised by the chat show host include messages that demonstrate that the social norms of American society are transgressed in this example of social life. These threads are:

- age differences;
- underage sex – statutory rape;
- destroying the morals of a minor;
- truancy – poor education;
- alcohol consumption by a minor;
- violence – exhibited against the boyfriend before the girl.

The conversation map created in this example comprises *interpersonal* (social network), *textual* (themes) and *ideational* (semantic network). In the semantic network shaped by the dialogue, the language carried ideas that are connected to other ideas. Consequently, other health concerns not specifically discussed by the group on stage may have been clear to the audience. These include risks to sexual health, risks of further pregnancies, and the risks of poor nutrition and obesity (the girl was grossly overweight at the age of fifteen).

This example takes us further into the links between the cultural, unconscious and concepts of acceptable societal behaviour, concepts of the young body and risk that this book is unable to pursue. These types of television programmes on risk topics, such as child abuse, sexual abuse and violence, prompt a formulation of response that is based on the embodied rationalities and irrationalities of otherness, desire, the emotions and the unconscious, which have their own, often non-linear, momentum and logic (Tulloch and Lupton 1997, 221). These televisual texts on health and to a large extent societal risk may be partly responded to on a subliminal level, involving what Tulloch and Lupton term 'message involvement', at a level of complexity that the audience may not be able to articulate but may well shape their decisions in constructing responses to risk which in turn is shaped through socio-cultural context.

The chat show, like some advertisements, presents as a form of commodification of risk. They both rely on images and storytelling as a process of communication. Many advertisers and chat show hosts try to sell us products or societal morality by playing on our weaknesses, vulnerabilities, vanities and fears thus generating the need for social compliance. They try to make us all obsessed with risks, even going as far as inventing new risks. It is this emotional and often unconscious response to bodily risk, as represented in the media and other forums, involving such strategies as projection, externalization and the return of the repressed, that may explain why some chat shows and advertisements attract so much attention when first screened and remain in people's memories.

Bands and travelling players

In Malawi in the late 1990s whilst on fieldwork I witnessed a form of risk communication that was quite outside my experience. A travelling band of players who were accompanied by a number of health promoters, were moving from village to village to inform the villagers about the risks of infectious diseases, including HIV, protection against malaria and seeking appropriate and timely care from health practitioners. Much of the way in which risk was communicated was through dance.

People's preconceived idea about dance is coloured by their exposure and in this culture dance is usually considered an elite art form. Professionals in psychology, education and health tend to think that dance is something which requires specific training that only a few talented artists can do; that it has nothing to do with education or medicine. We need to establish a different orientation about dance. In other cultures, like the indigenous peoples, dance is the most important form of education. Through it, value systems are passed on to the children, as are the most vital ways they deal with their mythology, speaking to their creator, blessing newborns and ushering the dying on safe journeys – all this is done through dance. Dance they believe is the most effective and holistic way of communicating with themselves and the higher powers (Halprin 2002).

From personal observations of dance in Malawian villages during 1991, it was clear that individuals were provided with considerable opportunity and capacity to delve into deep levels of knowledge in the body through movement and music that had not yet shifted into conscious awareness. The most extraordinary symbols were drawn out of their unconscious mental pictures, not realising where the images came from or what they were telling them until they danced it.

According to Halprin (cited in Barrett 1993) an important part of the process is to embody those images, using the body's language. This is different than trying to talk to the body using the rational mind. Word symbols are limited to our superficial knowledge of our world. Experiences from deeper layers do not have words. Yet, for Halprin (op. cit.) there is a movement experience that gives you a language for that image. You can connect with the feelings and make links to what the symbols mean in your life. When those dance and life themes connect that is when dance becomes significant, when it once again becomes a ritual. Dance movement provides a remarkable capacity to reflect what is happening internally, then to externalise and become conscious of it so that you can begin to make choices and change.

Another important part of the process is to have a witness, an objective observer of your ritual. If you have a witness who knows what you are doing in your dance, what your task is, they are able to keep you focused. The witness is a mirror, a support that intensifies the experience enabling you to press past that point of censure.

Barrett (op. cit.) cites Halprin's description of how in 'Circle the Earth' they worked with masks and internal warriors:

One young HIV-positive person drew a very powerful looking warrior who could confront anything and win. Yet when he went into his warrior stance to confront his fear saying 'I fear thee not,' his legs turned into spaghetti. He was so frightened he could barely move or breathe, his voice cracked. Yet the witness was there holding the warrior drawing saying you can do it. In that five minutes the young person's legs grew powerful and he was saying, 'I fear thee not,' from his guts and meant it. If there hadn't been a witness, chances are he would have retreated and given up. The movement reshaped itself and through it he developed a tool to find the strength in himself to overcome his fear.

Dance and drama takes a different form in the next example of communicating health risks to the public. In the following example from Canada, a young girl named Sara has a lot of things going on in her life and she is finding it hard to cope. In Canada, suicide accounts for 24 percent of all deaths among 15–24-year-olds and 16 percent among 16–44-year-olds as measured by WHO. Suicide is the second leading cause of death for Canadians between the ages of 10 and 24. The suicide rate for Canadians is 15 per 100 000 people. Yet, according to numerous studies, rates are even higher among specific groups. For example, the suicide rate for Inuit peoples living in Northern Canada is between 60 and 75 per 100 000 people, significantly higher than the general population (World Health Organization 2002).

Judith Marcuse Projects produced a dance performance entitled 'ICE: Beyond Cool' to address the problem of teen suicide by asking: Why do kids shut down and become 'cool'? The production was premiered in 1997 and a national tour took place in 2000. The production, based on three years of workshops conducted in Vancouver with more than 250 teenagers aged 15–18 years old, featured a 15-member cast of young professional actors and dancers from across Canada. Integrating dance, theatre, rock music and special effects, ICE was presented after-hours in shopping malls and arenas with a talkback session following each performance.

Case example: The ICE Project: Ice Beyond Cool (Marcuse 2000)

Produced by: DanceArts Vancouver; Artistic Director, Judith Marcuse

The main character is Sara, a young woman stressed out by having too much to do. Her parents are in the middle of a nasty divorce, a boy at her school has just committed suicide, her boyfriend is pressuring her to have sex and friends are pressuring her to try 'shrooms. Meanwhile, we learn that the boy she's supposed to be tutoring (another unwanted task that is just adding more stress) is experiencing his own problems. He appears at her house right after Sara has just had an argument with her mother about her rebellious behaviour. She is in no mood to deal with him and ends up yelling at him to go away. The next day at school, she learns that he was found dead the night before from a drug overdose.

Immediately, Sara blames herself and the fact that she had called him 'an asshole'. Through all this, it is gradually revealed that Sara's best friend, Chrissy, is experiencing her own problems, including an eating disorder and suicidal thoughts. Inner Sara believes it is for an adult to deal with but Sara doesn't want to lose her friend or end up feeling guilty. After a pivotal argument with her parents, she arrives at Chrissy's. It takes time, but they talk and eventually Chrissy feels better and Sara accepts the bottle of pills handed to her even though no promises were made between the two friends.

The play is interspersed throughout with dance scenes with a single character portraying feelings and emotions. There is also a musical interlude in which the players sing 'I hate my nose, I hate my chin, I hate my face, I hate my skin, I hate my zits, I hate my gut, I hate my tits, I hate my butt ...' The song is tongue-in-cheek but the message has just as much impact as the main story scenes.

'My life was portrayed with chilling accuracy.'

The Ice Project reported that after returning from the show, a teen confided to his mother that his friend was suicidal and that even he was having trouble with bullying at school. After realising how her own actions affected her children, a mother publicly vowed to go home and talk to her kids in a whole new way. A teacher left the show determined to lead the way in not shunning the loners and oddballs in her school.

The Report further highlighted what the audience said they had learned from the drama:

- more activism is needed within their communities;
- consumer hype has huge impact in their lives;
- schools are failing Canada's teens;
- the simple act of hugging can help immeasurably.

•it is very hard to find timely support, care and intervention. Waiting lists to get help are daunting;
• many disclosures of cluster health problems are not being adequately addressed, for example anorexia, depression, bi-polar disorder and bulimia;
• many feel out of control, with lives filled with stress and accelerating demands;
• the arts play a vital, important role in telling the truth and helping with the healing;
• small gestures, like a hug or a smile, can cut through despair and change a life;
• small, thoughtless actions and comments can hurt someone very deeply and have long-term effects;
• friends of at-risk youth are often sworn to secrecy and then get caught between being loyal and wanting to get adult help.

Health risk communication approaches, such as described above, fall into the category of empowerment, a concept developed by Paolo Freire (see for example Freire 1970). Empowerment theory suggests that a problem-posing process can help people overcome their sense of powerlessness, thus freeing them to make healthy choices. If members of a population (a) come together to see a dramatic presentation by group members in the form of role plays, stories, slides, photographs or songs; (b) participate actively in an open-ended problem-solving dialogue about those issues raised by the drama (by participating in a facilitated five-step process that includes asking individuals to describe what they see in the representation and what feelings it calls up; defining, as a group, the many levels of the problem; sharing similar experiences from their lives; questioning why this problem exists; and developing an action plan to address the problem); and (c) implement that action plan that addresses the problem at a community level, behaviour change will happen eventually. The most important result is permanent personal and community development.

Mapping for risk identification and communication

Again, built around the principles of his seminal work *Pedagogy of the Oppressed* (1970) and his subsequent books, Freire argues for a system of education that emphasises learning as an act of culture and freedom. He is best known for concepts such as 'conscientisation', a process by which the learner advances towards critical consciousness; 'dialectic', 'empowerment', 'generative themes/words', 'problematisation' and 'transformation of the world' are embedded in the processes of map-making for community communication purposes.

The way that people understand health risks is important in gaining their support for changing risky health behaviours or the environment in which such behaviours are fostered. If people believe that health is primarily a personal rather than social matter, then public-policy-oriented approaches are likely to be unsuccessful, while approaches reinforcing the responsibility of the individual will be favoured. The choice here is politically and socially critical because health as a personal matter assigns responsibility to individuals while policy-oriented approaches sees responsibility shared more equitably between government, the corporate world, the community and the individual.

Map-making is a form of communication that allows people to identify those aspects of their society and environment they think are important, and to represent the spatial relationships between those elements to others.

Geographic information systems (GIS) allow users to collect even larger amounts of data, which can be used later for both selective analysis and representation. Historically, these map-makers have been members of the scientific community, government officials, or workers with international agencies. In contrast, participatory mapping and participatory GIS (PGIS) attempt to give voice to community members in the language of maps, and to empower them in the collection and use of geographic data. Community members may take a small or large role in the map-making process. They may participate in data collection; provide information in the form of interviews or survey responses; produce hand-drawn maps; work with GIS to create, input or manage data; or become decision-makers regarding the collection, use or representation of that data.

Conclusion

Existing power structures can serve as a barrier to social change. Individuals or groups, who wish to undertake certain ameliorative action, often face resistance from social structures. For example, in India, caste, gender and class mediate the extent to which people can overcome restrictions and barriers to progress. Paradox and contradiction are also an integral part of the process of social change (Papa et al. 2000). Since established patterns of thought and behaviour are difficult to change, people often engage in an adjustment process until the new behaviour patterns are fully internalised.

In many countries around the world the rate of literacy is not very high; consequently we must also address the listening audience. When we invest in health risk communication we ensure a road to development through the media, that is, through radio and television, dramas and dance, storytelling and dialogue. Sustainability of development requires the institutionalisation of development communication. Future generations of health communicators need to be well informed about disparities in development so that they are able to create a media that has a positive holistic perspective of issues concerning health gender and human rights.

10 *Communication Shapes the World*

A cartoon sparks riots around the world. The Green Flag of Hammas changes the world in an afternoon. What we say about avian flu will impoverish thousands and perhaps save millions.

(Smith in Health e Communication Forum 2006)

Our perceptions of health risks and responses to them often seem inconsistent and perhaps irrational. Many health risks we perceive as great (such as the risk of brain cancer from cell phone use, or the risks associated with the spread of West Nile virus by mosquitoes) are often statistically far less likely to occur than more routine risks we face through our everyday behaviour (such as accidents from motor vehicle use or recreational activities). Over several generations, Western societies have incrementally developed a 'safety culture', that is, a culture that has instilled fears and an ever-diminishing tolerance for risks.

We tend to choose the type and number of dangers we worry about. Selection of our fears is influenced by a number of factors, including media bias, whether a given risk taps into our insecurities, offends our basic moral principles, or even permits criticism of disliked groups and institutions and provides symbols to attack or identify with; such may be the case in the context of mental ill health as discussed by Shula Ramon in Chapter 8.

It is a difficult and complex activity to communicate risk. Nicole West-Hayles (private communication 2006) comments that in Jamaica there are competing uncontrollable risk factors, such as issues of viable livelihoods and personal safety, that seem to be of greater importance than issues such as HIV/AIDS, avian flu, substance abuse, cancer or heart disease. In poor, urban communities, people see themselves more at risk of being shot first. There is an advertisement currently running on Jamaican radio that ends, 'Women stop protecting the gunmen.' But West-Hayes asks – How does she stop? Where is the safe home to go to? How does she leave this man without putting her family and herself at risk?

Risk perception research reveals that individuals typically find it difficult to evaluate expertise, and so they simplify. Individuals seem to pay more attention to what the potential consequences are than the probability of occurrence. Furthermore, once people perceive a potential risk, it becomes difficult to change that initial perception.

Individuals base their judgements about health risks on factors such as individual perception of risk, arising out of values and beliefs, converging with societal, political, cultural influences, religion, their knowledge, understanding and experience of the risk in question (Figure 10.1). These coalesce to form a platform from which individuals can make a decision concerning their behaviour. Of course, this is dependent upon their desire to change or indeed whether it is within their power to change. Moreover, when considering risk communication we also need to recognise a balance between three key areas of risk understanding (Figure 10.2): *objective calculation of risk* helps us understand some aspects of risk; our *subjective understanding* of risk based on our experience of the risk in question influences our decisions; and our *ability to live with uncertainty* pose real challenges for risk communication.

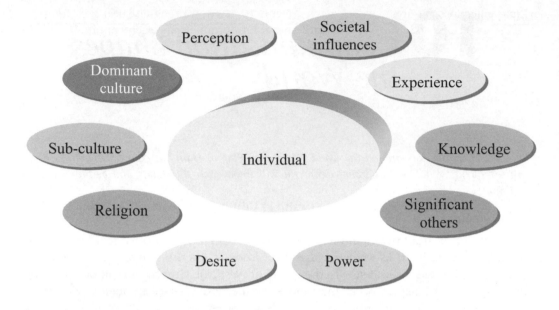

Figure 10.1   Influences that inform individual health risk decision-making

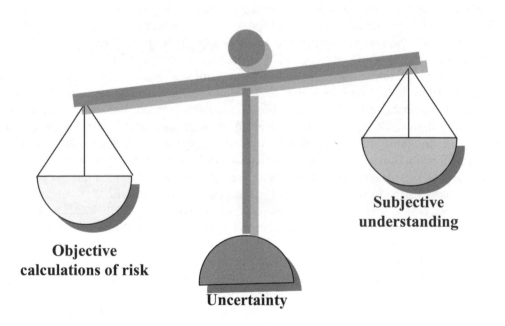

Figure 10.2   Risk communication requires a balance between three elements.

The collection of individual perspectives (Figure 10.3) is now brought to bear at community level. Depending upon cultural types, grid and group formulations, each community forms its own collective decisions concerning risk behaviour. So, if the risk concerns eating meat or extreme sports, the community forms a view on the level of acceptable risk.

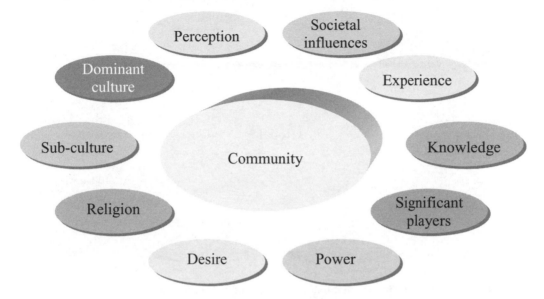

Figure 10.3   Community perspectives underpinning risk decision-making

Individual, community concerns begin to be overshadowed at societal level where health risk communication based on scientific data and population level public health concerns assume a political dimension (Figure 10.4).

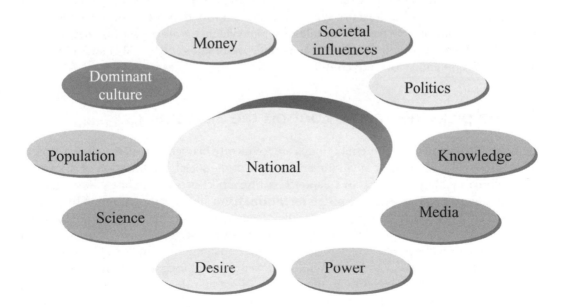

Figure 10.4   National considerations underpinning risk communication approaches

At the global level, the complexity of trans-governmental working is overlaid on national concerns and competing priorities (Figure 10.5).

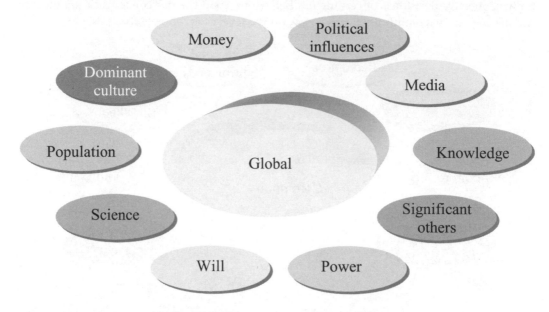

Figure 10.5   Global considerations that influence risk communication strategies

At the macro level, the model in Figure 10.6 demonstrates the complexity of influences that hamper or enhance the possibility of effective risk communication from the individual to the global level. Global concerns can directly impact on individuals and individuals can begin, through the power of the Internet, to have an influence at global levels.

We need to understand the decision-making process holistically. It is not primarily about what evidence we have, but how decisions are made, and why they are made in specific ways. Otherwise, we may run the risk of only talking about evidence while forgetting that decisions on the part of the individual, community, national governments and global organisations take a number of different factors into consideration.

He who picks the images controls the dialogue

The news media and environmental groups are frequently blamed for public overreaction to events such major oil spills or avian flu, an example of the social amplification of risk which was explored by Mary Northrop in Chapter 6. A disconnect between public views regarding the consequences and necessary remedies on the one hand and expert opinion on these same questions on the other is a frequently identified consequence of this phenomenon. A more comprehensive examination of the ways in which scientific messages can fail to inform the public or to rationalise public policy suggests however, that a more complex phenomenology is at work. Perceived risks can be attenuated as well as amplified, and many organisations besides the news media contribute to the shaping of public risk attitudes. As a result, social and political questions of blame can prove difficult to disentangle from scientific questions of impact.

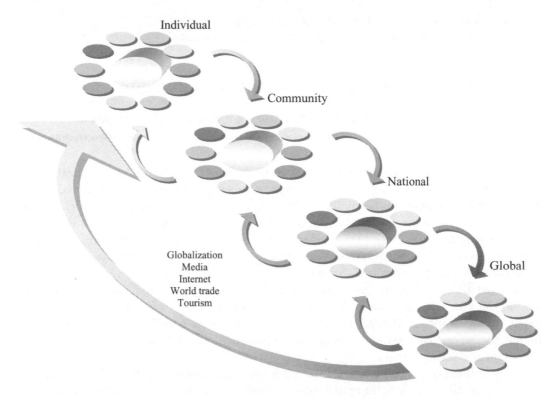

Figure 10.6 Interrelational context of risk communication prompting different styles and approaches to create effective and sustainable change

Tulloch and Lupton (1997, 221) suggest that media representation of health risks do not only involve the hierarchical steps of 'attracting awareness', 'understanding the message', 'identifying with the message', or 'assessing personal relevance' that are so often identified in the health communication literature. What is missing in this formulation of response are the embodied and the unconscious, which have their own, often non-linear, momentum and logic.

Although a multiplicity of theories and concepts have emerged during the past 50 years concerning health communication, they have fundamentally offered two different diagnoses and answers to the problem of health risk behaviour. While one position has argued that the problem was largely due to lack of information among individuals and populations, the other one suggested that power inequality was the underlying problem. Because the diagnoses were different, recommendations were different, too. Running the risk of over-generalisation, it could be said that theories and intervention approaches fell in different camps on the following points:

- cultural versus environmental explanations for underdevelopment;
- psychological versus socio-political theories and interventions;
- attitudinal and behavioural models versus structural and social models;
- individual- versus community-centred interventions development;
- hierarchical and sender-oriented versus horizontal and participatory communication models;

- active versus passive conceptions of audiences and populations;
- participation as means versus participation as end approaches.

Health risk communication – a changing paradigm

The voice of the people to the powerful, not only the voice of the powerful to the people.

(Smith 2006)

Walter Saba (Health e Communication Forum 2006) considers that health communication has changed dramatically over the past 40 years, passing from being initially a matter of production of simple print materials to becoming a vital strategic component of health programmes. This evolution, he believes, is characterised by a shift in paradigms over time. In the initial paradigm, emphasis was given to the impersonal promotion of health services assuming that people who know where the health services are located will find their way to clinics. Later, the emphasis switched to a more active approach emphasising outreach workers and community-based distributors. Third, in time came the social marketing paradigm, developed by the commercial concept that consumers will buy the products they want at subsidised prices. Today, we are in the era of behaviour change communication, based on behavioural science models for individuals, communities and organisations that emphasise the process of both individual and social change.

Each of these paradigms has had a special prominence during specific periods in history, however, they also co-exist at the present time and they all may be relevant and complementary to each other, depending on the expected results and underlying conditions of a particular setting.

At present, it seems that a new paradigm is emerging beyond the current behavioural change communication (BCC) model (see for example Prochaska and Velicer 1997; Prochaska, Redding and Evers 1997). This new paradigm considers that communication can influence not only individual behaviours, but also major determinants of poor health such as policies and practices that determine gender and social inequalities, can link health communication interventions to other social programmes, can promote effective leadership for health to foster public support for urgent health issues, and can forge partnerships between the private and public sectors to improve health conditions at all levels of society.

The emergence of such a new paradigm would have major consequences on the reasons to invest in health communication as well as in the measurement of its impact. Saba (Health e Communication Forum 2006) would call the new paradigm an 'integrated approach to health communication', because it opens without restrictions the boundaries of the field of health communication to knowledge and practices from different sciences and disciplines such as economics, social sciences, cultural studies, marketing and others.

The integrated approach recognises that behavioural and social change are complex matters and, as such, they are the result of a combination of factors. Because these factors have different causes, it is likely that they will respond to different interventions and not to the same intervention all the time. That is why the approach calls for an integration of tactics and strategies, because it acknowledges the special contribution of each intervention to influence specific factors and the need to put different interventions together depending on the complexity of the health problem. It recognises that all the factors affecting people's poor health cannot be significantly affected by one intervention alone (for example, social mobilisation). Integration recognises the need to unite and the need for diversity, joining with something else that will make health risk communication interventions more powerful, leaving behind old myths and prejudices. Villalobos (Health e Communication Forum 2006) illustrates this point from a Peruvian perspective where health risks are communicated by traditional dances like marinera, musica andina, autochthonic languages like Quechua, Aymara and so on. Cultural forms are used because people receive and remember them better than the technical language of the professional.

Health risk communication offers a unique platform for strategic planning and action to foster individual and social change. Its uniqueness relies precisely on the fact that its practice is nourished by knowledge from several sciences and arts; knowledge that otherwise would be fragmented and dispersed. This confluence of knowledge becomes systemic only because it can be articulated in health communication theory and practice (Saba in Health e Communication Forum 2006).

For every complicated question there is a simple and incorrect answer

Strategic health communication accepts all forms of communication as valid and tries to define what is needed to accomplish a specific goal. Smith (2006 Health e Communication Forum), suggests that, for example, to inform people that a tsunami is on the way, grassroots communication would not be an ideal choice, neither would attempting to convince people that a new vaccine does not kill children using a pamphlet. Attempting to change the lifestyle of millions of overweight, confused and marketed-oriented Americans so that they eat and exercise in a way that produces healthy reductions in high Body Mass Index (BMI) via motivational TV advertisements may not be an appropriate vehicle. However, introducing a change to national policy on the cost of AIDS drugs using grassroots communication approaches would be a very important part of that strategy.

One critical weakness in the practice of much of the health risk communication profession is the reliance on intermediate indicators of success, such as changes in knowledge, attitudes and even behaviour. However, if knowledge of HIV and AIDS in Africa, for example, is high why does the infection continue to spread? Clearly, the plethora of multisectoral players in the response to the pandemic in most of Africa and elsewhere has achieved an initial level of information effects. There is, however, a further step which should be taken to push for a deeper level of knowledge, understanding and bring communities face-to-face with the need for, and commitment to, behavioural change.

Both theoretically and practically health communication professionals need to discuss and agree upon a common language, even before we discuss what is the dominant model driving the field. For instance, as long as information is misunderstood as communication, we will continue to see many public health programmes focusing attention on producing 'information materials' to educate or inform the public. Based on research and project officers' experiences, at least of large-scale health projects, communication is still operating at the information, consultation and at times collaboration level. Rarely do we see an entirely citizen-controlled communication effort and thus the theoretical trends in health communication do not seem to follow very closely to what is practiced. It is often assumed that services are in place and accessible to the population and as health communication serves a supportive role to services, it cannot be very effective if there are no services. Health communication without services discredits communicators and audiences can lose trust in the message. (This is one problem in using mass media that cannot distinguish between audiences who have access to services and those who do not.)

The moment health communication is equated with information we are bound to face resistance from donors and management that decide the budgets, because rarely would providing information alone translate into an improved health outcome. On the other hand, participatory communication takes much more time and in doing so generally loses out to other approaches that take less time. If participatory approaches demonstrate impact through qualitative research and focus principally on impact as valued by those they are designed to benefit, they generally lose out to approaches that can quantify impact in terms that are most valued by those who have funded the initiative.

Often expediency determines health risk communication decisions, and trumps evidence. This is why what is easy, cheap and fast is preferred over integrated strategies. Because communication resources are limited and the number of staff insufficient to the task, decision makers need quick and dirty solutions to what they perceive are the real problems. Moreover, since politicians and donor agencies like high-profile media events, health communication people have pressures to produce something by tomorrow. This is why short-term thinking and decisions predominates over what we know usually works better. In this scenario there is an inbuilt tendency to invest in results that can be measured and in impact measures that are easily achievable with early results. Consequently, mass-media campaigns, media events, press releases and the like predominate and are expected from health communication personnel. But for all the many cruel lessons that the AIDS pandemic should teach the health communication community, and those who should support it, there is one that stands out: what appeared to work over three years had little impact over five or ten; and what worked over five, ten or 15 years would have been very difficult to quantify over three years. We have a collective responsibility to develop strategies that have long-term impact.

Thus, unless we clearly communicate to the policy makers, media and other professionals what can and cannot be achieved by health risk communication, we may all continue to argue over the same issues every few years and in turn not be able to move the field forward. We need, therefore, to be clear about our terms. We talk a lot about evidence and impact, but we need to define what we mean. What matters is what lasts – impact over what period, according to whom, leaving behind what capacity? What does an integrated strategic health communication initiative mean? Too often it turns out to be a mass-media campaign with a participatory component to it, still based in essence in getting a series of messages to people rather than providing channels to get messages from them (Deane in Health e Communications Forum 2006).

Facts are no competition for emotive messages today

The business of selling fear is pervasive and has been enhanced by the emergence of the Internet. The media plays an important role in informing the public of health and environmental risks, but the quality and accuracy of reporting on issues is not guaranteed, and is biased toward sensational and dramatic stories. Fear is a common side effect.

The reality gap between the facts about so-called pandemics such as bird flu, SARS or foot and mouth disease and the politicised public reaction to it has left us with a confused and dangerous mess of a situation where, in the UK, policy seems to be run in tandem by two old

BBC sitcom characters from *Dad's Army* simultaneously shouting 'Don't Panic!' and 'We're Doomed!'.

In the context of the contemporary concerns surrounding avian flu, Hume (2006) claims that the British Government has tried to hold the line against hysteria and appear reasonable, issuing a new 'don't panic' message. The message, however, is being repeatedly subverted by opposition politicians, experts, campaigners and media voices accusing the Government of complacency or a cover-up, and demanding more and more precautionary measures. In this, Hume (op. cit.) argues that New Labour has made a rod for its own back, by institutionalising the precautionary principle at the heart of Government policy on everything from food dye to mobile phones, and by emphasising the need to reduce risk on every front. Now, fearful of being accused of not intervening enough to prevent a potential threat to public health, the Government's response is to up the ante further, to try to demonstrate that it is fully prepared.

Given that producing fear is easier than diminishing it, how should we manage public fears? Part of the answer lies in the development of trust. We need to develop and maintain trust, and cultivate respect in institutions. For this, we need to examine history and the roots of trust. Since the early 1980s, trust in Western government institutions has fallen. But although trust in government is low, public expectation of its responsibility for the protection of health and the environment remains high. Conflicting conclusions from different scientific studies contribute to public scepticism and to speculation about conflicts of interest related to the sources of funding.

Consultation and communication with the public can help garner trust in public institutions. Public participation in decision-making can contribute to this cause, as well as involving experts skilled at communicating risks. Finally, if we are to reduce the fearful aspect of our various cultures around the world, we also need to learn from our mistakes – to examine history to look at instances where trust in government was lost.

Media can play a significant role: raising awareness of the issues within government and civil society, engaging civil society in debate, interrogating policy and debating alternatives, promoting transparency in policy making and implementation, and building political commitment to inclusive communication policies. However, at present media do not generally have the capacity to play this role. Few journalists and editors are familiar enough with the issues to report and analyse them effectively and communication is not seen as a priority for coverage.

What is really important to remember is that the world is globalising. Health risks exist for those intrepid travellers as well as tourists, it exists for those who remain in their own countries – from people and animals and birds who bring infectious or chemical or indeed nuclear agents to us. We need to be aware of the issues that are submerged below the surface that impact on decision-making regarding health risk behaviours globally – and develop a language or languages in which we can communicate health risk globally.

However, we must also be aware that taking risks is inevitable and in many cases, necessary for life. We take risks every day and mostly we do not pause to calculate the odds of something harmful happening. For some taking risks with their health is an important part of their recovery process; for example, in mental health, living in the community may well pose a risk to the individual from other people who are fearful of them, but it is an important step for the individual concerned to re-integrate into the community. For others, the risks associated with taking specific drug therapies are perhaps less than those of not taking the drugs.

Although people may be somewhat aware of health risks, few understand how, or why, such risks fit into their lives. An investigation into their perceptions may well reveal not only a lack of comprehension, but also an image of risk communicators as remote, dispassionate and unapproachable. This image is often inadvertently perpetuated by alarmist, brusque and confusing messages that further distance individuals.

We know that communities vary in norms, values, beliefs, practices, cultural traditions and so on, therefore, we may need intermediate to long-term grassroots qualitative and quantitative research, to enable us to derive information for the design of culturally sensitive, community-appropriate and effective health communication strategies, with appropriate indices to monitor and measure success.

Challenges

If participatory approaches that involve communities and their structures, with local stakeholders, in all aspects of health risk communication can succeed and justify the necessary investment, then there are some pertinent questions to ask.

- To what extent are target/affected communities involved in all aspects of problem identification, prioritisation and the development of (funded) programmes that are meant to address health problems?
- How conducive are political and socio-economic environments? How widespread are they in the developing world? What effect do they have on success?
- How much donor interest is there to provide sufficient resources?
- How patient are policy makers and donors to wait to see change?
- How committed are donors and NGOs to long-term communication efforts until changes emerge at community level?
- To what extent are donor/NGO and governments/political partnerships in health communications devoid of mutual suspicion?

In conclusion

This book has attempted to draw together a number of significant factors that impact on communicating health risks to the public. We have journeyed from a global perspective in which we explored risk generically, moving to viewing risk from the global village in Chapter 2. In Chapter 3 we explored the cultural meaning of risk before leading into a discussion of risk perception in Chapter 4 by Woody Caan and Dawn Hillier. Our journey continued as we delved into the art and science of risk communication in Chapter 5 and unpacked through examples the issues surrounding the social amplification, attenuation and impact, in the case of sexual health, of risk through communication styles and approaches. Andy Stevens focused on youth resilience as he explored the ways in which fast cars and cool cigarettes portrayed in the media impacted on young people. In Chapter 8, Shula Ramon invited us to consider the role of the media in the context of mental health. In Chapter 9, I presented what I consider to be the social life of risk communication through the genre of storytelling in fairy tales and soap operas among other cultural forms. Finally, this chapter has focused on the question of how risk communication shapes the world in which we live and I would like to repeat Smith's (Health e Communications Forum 2006) comment:

> *Communication shapes the world. A cartoon sparks riots around the world. The Green Flag of Hammas changes the world in an afternoon. What we say about avian flu will impoverish thousands and perhaps save millions.*

Bibliography

Adams, J. and White, M. (2005), 'When the Population approach to Prevention Puts the Health of Individuals at Risk', *International Journal of Epidemiology* 34, 40–43.

Adler, N. J. (1997), *International dimensions of organizational behaviour*, 3rd edn (Cincinnati, OH: Shout-Western College Publishing).

Agyepong, I. A., Aryee, B., Dzikunu, H. and Manderson, L. (1995), 'Chapter 4 Community Perceptions of Malaria', *The Malaria manual: Guidelines for the rapid assessment of social, economic and cultural aspects of malaria*, UNDP/World Bank/WHO Special Programme for Research & Training in Tropical Diseases (Switzerland: WHO).

Agyepong, I. A. (1992), 'Malaria: Ethnomedical perceptions and practice in an Adangme farming community and implications for malaria control', *Social Science and Medicine* 35:2, 131–137.

Agyepong, I. A. and Manderson, L. (1999), 'Malaria prevention in the Greater Accra Region, Ghana: Mosquito avoidance and bed net use in the greater Accra region, Ghana', *Journal of Biosocial Science* 31:1, 79–92.

Ahorlu, C. K., Dunyo, S. K., Afari, E. A., Koram, K.A., Nkrumah, F. K. (1997), 'Malaria-related beliefs and behaviour in southern Ghana: implications for treatment, prevention and control', *Tropical Medicine and International Health* 2:5, 488–499.

Anderson, C. A. (1983), 'Imagination and Expectation: The Effect of Imagining Behavioral Scripts on Personal Intentions', *Journal of Personality and Social Psychology* 45:2, 293–305.

Andreasen, A. R. (1995), *Marketing social change: changing behavior to promote health, social development, and the environment* (San Francisco: Jossey-Bass).

Appardurai, A. (1990), 'Disjuncture and Difference in the Global Cultural Economy', *Public Culture* 2:2, 1–24.

Arnett, J. (2002), 'Developmental sources of crash risk in young drivers', *Injury Prevention* 8, 17–23.

Ashton, C. H. (1986), 'Adverse Effects of Prolonged Benzodiazepine Use', *Adverse Drug Reaction Bulletin* 118, 440–443.

—— (2002), 'Benzodiazepine Abuse', in Caan, A. W. and de Belleroche, J. (eds), *Drink, Drugs and Dependence* (Routledge), Ch. 15 197–211.

—— (2004), 'Protracted withdrawal symptoms from benzodiazepines', in Miller, N. (ed.) *Comprehensive Handbook of Drug & Alcohol Addiction* (Informa Healthcare).

Ausems, M., Mesters, van Breukelen, I. and De Vries, G. (2003), 'Do Dutch 11-12 years olds who never smoke, smoke experimentally or smoke regularly have different demographic backgrounds and perceptions of smoking?', *European Journal of Public Health* 13:2, 160–167.

Bailey, C. and Pang, T. (2004), 'Healthy Information for all by 2015?', *The Lancet* 364, 224.

Bakewell, J. (2006), 'At risk of offending you', *The Independent*, 20 January 2006.

Bandura, A. (1977a), Social Learning Theory (New York: Prentice–Hall).

—— (1977b), *Self-Efficacy: The Exercise of Control* (New York: Freeman).

Barke, R., Jenkins-Smith, H., Slovic, P. (1997), 'Risk perceptions of men and women scientists', *Social Science Quarterly* 78, 167–76.

Barrett, S. (1993), 'Dance as Healing Communication – an inner view with Anna Halprin', published in Healing Health Care Communications, www.mysticmolecules.com/articles/Halprin-DanceAsHealing.pdf.

Bauman, Z. (2002), *Society Under Siege* (Polity Press: Cambridge).

—— (2003), *Liquid Love: On the Frailty of Human Bonds* (Cambridge: Polity Press).

Baume, C., Helitzer, D. and Kachur, S. P. (2000), 'Patterns of care for childhood malaria in Zambia', *Social Science and Medicine* 25, 277–292.

Bazerman, M. H. and Watkins, M. D. (2004), *Predictable Surprises: The Disasters you Should Have Seen Coming, and How to Prevent Them* (Boston: Harvard Business School Press).

Bazerman, M. H., Messick, D. M., Tenbrunsel, A. E. and Wade-Benzoni K. A. (eds) (1997), *Environment, ethics, and behaviour* (San Francisco: New Lexington), 277–313. Revised version in *The University of Chicago Legal Forum* 1997, 59–99.

Barzani, B. (2006) 'Bird Flu, Kurdistan' (forthcoming), www.kurdmedia.com/articles.asp?id=11064

BBC News World Service 31 October 2005 <http://news.bbc.co.uk/1/hi/world/africa/3969693.stm> (viewed January 2005).

BBC (2005), 'US "harming" Uganda's Aids battle' <http://news.bbc.co.uk/go/pr/fr/-/1/hi/world/africa/4195968.stm>

Beal, B. (1995), 'Disqualifying the official: An exploration of social resistance through the subculture of skateboarding', *Sociology of Sport Journal* 12, 252–67.

Becher, H. (2001),'Smoking prevalence and cigarette consumption', in Boreham, R. and Shaw, A. (eds).

Beck, U. (1992), *Risk Society: Towards a New Modernity* (London: Sage).

Beck, U. (1999), *What Is Globalization?* (Cambridge: Polity Press).

Beck, V., Huang, G. C., Pollard, W. E., Johnson, T. J. (2003), 'Telenovela viewers and health information', paper presented at the American Public Health Association 131st Annual Meeting and Exposition (San Francisco, California).

Becker, H. (1995), *Namibian Women's Movement 1980-1992* (Frankfurt: Verlag fuer Interkulturelle Kommunikation).

Bentall, R. (2004), *Madness Explained: Psychosis and Human Nature* (London: Allen Lane).

Bernhardt, J. M., (2004), 'Communication at the Core of Effective Public Health', *American Journal of Public Health* 94:12, 2051–2053.

Bernstein, P. L. (1999), 'Facing The Consequences', *Economics and Portfolio Strategy*, 1 October (New York: Peter L. Bernstein, Inc).

Boreham, R. and Shaw, A. (eds) (2001), *Smoking, drinking and drug use among young people in England in 2000* (DoH).

Bourdieu, P. (1986), 'The forms of capital', in Baron, S., Field, J. and Schuller, T. (eds), *Social Capital: Critical Perspectives* (Oxford: Oxford University Press).

—— (1990), *In Other Words: Essays Towards a Reflexive Sociology* (Cambridge: Polity Press).

Boyle, M. (2002), *Schizophrenia: A Scientific Delusion?* 2nd edn (London: Routledge).

Bradley, D. (1991), 'Malaria – whence and whither', in Targett, G. A. T. (ed.), *Malaria: waiting for the vaccine* (New York: John Wiley & Sons).

Brain, J. B. (1990), ' "But only we black men die": the 1929–1933 malaria epidemics in Natal and Zululand'. *Contree: Journal of South African Urban and Regional History* 27, 18–25.

Breakwell, G. M. and Barnett, J. (2001), 'The Impact of Social Amplification on Risk Communication', *Contract Research Report 322/2001* (London, Sudbury: Health and Safety Executive).

Breman, J. G. and Campbell, C. C. (1988), 'Combating severe malaria in African children', *Bulletin of the World Health Organization* 66:5, 611–20.

Bricker, J., Leroux, B., Peterson, A., Kealey, K., Sarason, I., Andersen, M. and Marek, P. (2003), 'Nine-year prospective relationship between parental smoking cessation and children's daily smoking'. *Addiction* 98:5, 585–593.

Bristow, J. (2005), 'Unwrapping the "cotton wool" kids', Spiked Risk, www.spiked-online.com/articles/0000000CAAFF.htm

Brunn, S. D. and Leinback, T. R. (1991), *Collapsing Space and Time: Geographic Aspects of Communications and Information* (London: Harper Collins Academic).

Burke, K. (1945), *A Grammar of Motives* (Berkeley, CA: University of California Press).

Burns, W., Slovic, P., Kasperson, R., Kasperson, J., Renn, O., and Emani, S. (1990), *Social amplification of risk: An empirical study* (Carson City, NV: Nevada Agency for Nuclear Projects Nuclear Waste Project Office).

Butt, L. (2005), ' "Lipstick Girls" And "Fallen Women":AIDS And Conspiratorial Thinking In Papua', *Indonesia Cultural Anthropology* 20:3, 412–442, ISSN 0886-7356, electronic ISSN 1548-1360.

Caan, A. W. (1991), 'Preliminary observations on a drugs and AIDS initiative for prisoners in the South West Thames health region', *British Journal of Addiction* 86, 1516.

Carroll. J. S. (1978), 'The effect of imagining an event on expectations for the event: An interpretation in terms of the availability heuristic', *Journal of Experimental Social Psychology* 14, 88–96.

Cassell, M. M., Jackson, C. and Cheuvront, B. (1998), 'Health Communication on the Internet: An Effective Channel for Health Behavior Change?', *Journal of Health Communication* 3:1, 71–79.

Centre for International Forestry Research (CIFOR) (2003), 'Livestock Development and Deforestation Brazil's Amazon', News Online No. 33, www.cifor.cgiar.org/docs/_ref/publications/newsonline/33/livestock.htm (accessed 05/11/2005).

Center for Risk Communication (2001), www.centerforriskcommunication.com/home.htm.

Chaiken, S. and Trope, Y. (1999), *Dual-process theories in social psychology* (New York: Guilford).

CIFOR (2003), 'Science for Forests and People', *CIFOR Annual Report 2003*.

Ciompi, L. (1980), 'Catamnestic long-term study on the course of life and aging of schizophrenics', *Schizophrenia Bulletin* 6, 606–618.

Clarke, D. D., Ward, P. J. and Truman, W. A. and Bartle, C. (2002), 'Sequential case-study of police road accident files involving young drivers, motorcycles or work-related accidents', in proceedings of *Behavioural Research in Road Safety: Twelfth Seminar* (London: Department for Transport), ISBN 1 85112 593 0, pp. 16–35.

Clifford, J. (1997), *Routes: travel and translation in the late twentieth century* (Cambridge: Harvard University Press).

Cooper, D., Atkins, F. and Gillen, D. (2005), 'Measuring the impact of passenger restrictions on new teenage drivers', *Accident Analysis & Prevention* 37:1, 19–23.

Corrao, M., Guidon, G., Sharma, N. and Shokoohi, D. (2000), *Tobacco Control Profiles* (Atlanta: American Cancer Society).

Crouch, E. A. C. and Wilson, R., (eds) (1981), *Risk/benefit analysis* (Cambridge, MA: Ballinger).

Cosio-Zavala, M. E. and Gastineau, B. (1997), *Women and Families: Changes in the Status of Women as a Factor and a Consequence of Changes in Family Dynamics* (Paris: Committee for the International Cooperation in Research in Demography).

Coupland, D. M. (1991), *Generation X: Tales for an accelerated culture* (first published by St Martin's Press: USA 1991; London: Abacus 1992).

Covello, V. T. (1998), 'Risk perception, risk communication, and EMF exposure: Tools and techniques for communicating risk information', in Matthes, R., Bernhardt, J. H., Repacholi, M. H. (eds) 'Risk Perception, Risk Communication, and Its Application to EMF Exposure', Proceedings of the *World Health Organization/ICNRP International Conference (ICNIRP 5/98)* (Vienna, Austria: International Commission on Non-Ionizing Radiation Protection) 1998, 179–214.

Covello, V. T., Slovic, P. and von Winterfeldt, D. (1986), 'Risk Communication: A Review of the Literature', *Risk Abstracts* 3:4, 172–182.

Covello, V. T., McCallum, D. B. and Pavlova, M. T. (eds) (1989), *Effective Risk Communication: The Role and Responsibility of Government and Nongovernment Organizations* (New York, NY: Plenum Press).

—— 'Principles and guidelines for improving risk communication', ibid. pp. 3–16.

Covello, V. T., Peters, R. G., Wojtecki, J. G. and Hyde, R. C. (2001), 'Risk Communication, the West Nile Virus Epidemic, and Bioterrorism: Responding to the Communication Challenges Posed by the Intentional or Unintentional Release of a Pathogen in an Urban Setting', *Journal of Urban Health: Bulletin of the New York Academy of Medicine* 78:2, 382–391, June 2001.

Covello, V. T. and Sandman, P. M. (2001), 'Risk communication: Evolution and revolution', in Wolbarst, A. (ed.) *Solutions to an Environment in Peril* (Baltimore, MD: John Hopkins University Press), 164–178.

Cutter, S. L. (1993), *Living with risk* (London: Edward Arnold).

Cvetkovich, G. and Earle, T.C. (eds) (1991), 'Risk and Psychology: Special Issue', *Journal of Cross-Cultural Psychology* 22, 1.

—— (1992), 'Environmental hazards and the public', in Cvetkovich, G. and Earle, T.C. (eds) 'Public reactions to environmental hazards', *Journal of Social Issues* 48:4, 1–20.

Cvetkovich, G., Earle, T. C., Schinke, S. P., Gilchrist, L. D. and Trimble, J. E. (1987), 'Child and adolescent drug use: A judgment and information processing perspective to health-behavior interventions', *Journal of Drug Education* 17, 295–313.

D'Adesky, A-C. (2004), *Moving mountains: the race to treat global AIDS* (London: Verso).

Dale, S. (April 2003), 'Preventing Pesticide Poisonings in Ecuador: Integrated pest management yields economic and health benefits', Health an Ecosystem Approach: The International Development Research Centre, www.idrc.ca/ecohealth (accessed 12 September 2005).

Damasio, A. R. (1994), *Descartes' error: Emotion, reason, and the human brain* (New York: Avon).

Dake, K. (1991), 'Orienting dispositions in the perception of risk: an analysis of contemporary worldviews and cultural biases', *Journal of Cross-Cultural Psychology* 22, 61–82.

Davidson, L. (2003), *Living Outside Mental Illness: Qualitative Studies of Recovery in Schizophrenia* (New York: New York University Press).

Davison, C, Davey Smith, G. and Frankel S. (1991), 'Lay epidemiology and the prevention paradox', *Sociology of Health and Illness* 13, 1–19.

Davison, C., Frankel, S. and Smith, G. D. (1992), 'The Limits of Popular Lifestyle: Re-assessing "fatalism" in the Popular Culture of Illness Prevention', *Social Science & Medicine* 34:6, 675–685.

Deegan, P. (1996), 'Recovery form a journey of the heart', *Psychiatric Rehabilitation Journal* 19, 91–97.

Delaney, A., Lough, B., Whelan, M. and Cameron, M. (2004) *A review of Mass Media Campaigns in Road Safety* (Monash Univ. Australia).

Department of Health (DoH) (1998), *Smoking Kills: A White Paper on Tobacco* (London: SO).

—— (2002), *Statistics on smoking cessation services in health authorities: England, April to September 2001* (DoH).

—— (2004), *Choosing Health: Making healthy choices easier* (London: HMSO).

Department for Transport (DfT) (2002), *Behavioural Research in Road Safety 12th Report* (London: HMSO).

—— (2004), *Behavioural Research in Road Safety 14th Report* (London: HMSO).

Dobson, A., Brown, W., Ball, J., McFadden, M. and Walker, M. (2000), *Female driver behaviour and road crash involvement* (Canberra: Australian Transport Safety Bureau).

Doherty, S., Andrey, J. and McGregor, C. (1998), 'The situational risks of young drivers: the influence of passengers, time of day and day of the week on accident rates', *Accident Analysis and Prevention* 30, 45–52.

Doniger, W. and Kakar, S. (2002), *Vastsayana Kama Sutra: A New Translation* (Oxford: Oxford University Press).

Double, D. (2005), 'Paradigm Shift in Psychiatry', in Ramon, S. and Williams. J .E. (eds) *Mental Health at the Crossroad: The Promise of the Psychosocial Approach* (Aldershot: Ashgate Publishing), pp. 65–80.

Douglas, M. (1966), *Purity and Danger: An Analysis of Concepts of Pollution and Taboo* (London: Routledge and Kegan Paul).

—— (1992), *Risk and Blame: Essays in Cultural Theory* (London: Routledge).

Douglas, M. and Wildavsky, A. (1982), *Risk and Culture: An Essay on the Selection of Technical and Environmental Dangers* (University of California Press).

Ebanks, G. E. (1985), *Mortality, Fertility and Family Planning in Dominica and Saint Lucia* (London, Ontario, Canada: University of Western Ontario).

Elkind, D. (1967), 'Egocentrism in adolescence', *Child Development* 38, 1025–1034.

Epinge, S. (2003) 'The Relationship Between Gender Roles and HIV Infection in Namibia', in Otaala, B. (ed.) *HIV/AIDS: Government Leaders in Namibia Responding to the HIV/AIDS Epidemic* (Windhoek: University of Namibia Press).

Epstein, S. (1994), 'Integration of the cognitive and the psychodynamic unconscious'. *American Psychologist* 49, 709–724.

Erev, I. (1998), 'Signal detection by human observers: A cutoff reinforcement learning model of categorization decisions under uncertainty', *Psychological Review* 105, 280–298.

Espino, F., Manderson, L., Acuin, C., Domingo, F., Ventura, E. (1997), 'Perceptions of malaria in a low endemic area in the Philippines: transmission and prevention of disease', *Acta Tropica* 63, 221–239.

Evans, K. (2002), 'Taking Control of their Lives? Agency in Young Adult Transitions in England and the New Germany', *Journal of Youth Studies* 5:3, 245–269.

Fagan, P., Brook, J., Rubenstone, E. and Zhang, C. (2005), 'Parental occupation, education, and smoking as predictors of offspring tobacco use in adulthood: A longitudinal study', *Addictive Behaviors* 30:3, 517–529.

Fetherstonhaugh, D., Slovic, P., Johnson, S. M., and Friedrich, J. (1997), 'Insensitivity to the value of human life: A study of psychophysical numbing', *Journal of Risk and Uncertainty* 14:3, 282–300.

Finucane, M. L., Slovic, P., Mertz, C. K., Flynn, J., and Satterfield, T. A. (2000), 'Gender, race, perceived risk: The "white male" effect', *Health, Risk, & Society* 2, 159–172.

Fischer, S. (2005), 'Changing Culture Poses Health Risk in North', *At Guelph* 49:7

Fischhoff, B., Slovic, P., Lichtenstein, S. (1978), 'Fault trees: sensitivity of assessed failure probabilities to problem representation', *J Exp Psychol Hum Percept Perform* 4, 330–44.

Fischhoff, B., Slovic, P., Lichtenstein, S., Read, S., and Combs, B. (1978), 'How safe is safe enough? A psychometric study of attitudes towards technological risks and benefits', *Policy Sciences* 9, 127–152.

Fischhoff, B., Watson, S., Hope, C. (1984), 'Defining risk', *Policy Sciences* 17, 123–39.

Fischhoff, B., Svenson, O. (1988), 'Perceived risk of radionuclides: understanding public understanding', in Harley, J. H., Schmidt, G. D., Silini, G. (eds), *Radionuclides in the food chain* (Berlin: Springer-Verlag), 453–71.

Fischhoff, B. (1995), 'Risk perception and communication unplugged: Twenty years of progress', *Risk Analysis* 15:2, 137–145.

Fischhoff, B. and Downs, J. S. (1997), 'Communicating Foodborne Disease Risk', *Emerging Infectious Diseases* 3:4.

Fishbein, M. and Ajzen, I. (1975), *Belief, attitude, intention, and behavior: An introduction to theory and research* (Reading, MA: Addison-Wesley).

Flynn, J., Slovic, P., and Mertz, C. K. (1994), 'Gender, race, and perception of environmental health risks', *Risk Analysis* 14:6, 1101–1108.

Foster, S. (1995), 'Treatment of malaria outside the formal health services', *Journal of Tropical Medicine and Hygiene* 98: 29–34.

Friedman, T. (1999), *The Lexus and the Olive Tree* (London: Harper Collins).

Freire, P. (1970), *Pedagogy of the Oppressed* (Harmondsworth, Middlesex: Penguin).

Furedi, F. (2002), *The Culture of Fear, Risk Taking and the Morality of Low Expectation* (London: Continuum).

—— (2005), 'The Market in fear', Spiked Essays 26 September, www.spiked-online.com/printable/0000000CAD7B.htm.

Galavotti, C., Cabral, R. J., Lansky, A., Grimley, D. M., Riley, G. E., Prochaska, J. O. (1995), 'Validation of measures of condom and other contraceptive use among women at high risk for HIV infection and unintended pregnancy', *Health Psychology* 14:6, 570–578.

Galanti, M., Rosendahl, I., Post, A.. and Gilljam, H. (2001), 'Early gender differences in adolescent tobacco use – The experience of a Swedish cohort', *Scandinavian Journal of Public Health* 29:4, 314–317.

Garfinkel, H. (1956), 'Conditions of Successful Degredation Ceremonies', *American Journal of Sociology* 61, 420–4.

Giddens, A. (1990), *The Consequences of Modernity* (Cambridge: Polity).

—— (1991), *Modernity and self-identity* (Cambridge: Polity).

Gifford, S. (1986), 'The meaning of lumps: a case study of the ambiguities of risk', in Stall, R., Janes, C., Gifford, S. (eds), *Anthropology and epidemiology. Interdisciplinary approaches to the study of health and disease* (Dordrecht: Reidel Publishing).

Gigli, S. (2004), 'Children, Youth and Media Around the World: An Overview of Trends & Issues', InterMedia Survey Institute, for *UNICEF 4th World Summit on Media for Children and Adolescents*, Rio de Janeiro, Brazil, April 2004 .

Gilovich, T., (ed.) (1993), *How we know what isn't so* (New York: Free Press).

Glantz, S. A., Kacirk, K. W., McCulloch, C. (2004), 'Back to the future: Smoking in movies in 2002 compared with 1950 levels', *Am. J Public Health* 94: 261–263.

Global Youth Tobacco Survey Collaborative Group (GYTS) (2002), 'Tobacco use among youth: a cross country comparison', *Tobacco Control* 11, 252–270.

Goffman, I. (1961), *Asylums* (Penguin, Harmondsworth).

Green, E. C. (1998), *Indigenous theories of contagious disease* (Walnut Creek: Altamira Press).

Gregerson, S. and Berg, H. (1994), 'Lifestyle and accidents among young drivers', *Accident Analysis and Prevention* 26, 297–303.

Gregory, W. L., Cialdini, R. B. and Carpenter, K. M. (1982), 'Relevant scenarios as mediators of likelihood estimates and compliance: Does imagining make it so?', *Journal of Personality and Social Psychology* 43, 89–99.

Griffiths, R. (1994), 'Call for action on men's health', *Annual report of West Midland Regional Director of Public Health* (Birmingham: West Midlands Regional Health Authority).

Harding, C. M., Brooks, G. W., Asologa, Y., Brier, A. (1987), 'The Vermont Longitudinal Studies of Persons with Severe Mental Illness', *American Journal of Psychiatry* 144, 718–726.

Halpin, T. (2005), 'Children must learn to embrace risk, heads are told', *Times Online*, www.timesonline.co.uk/newspaper/0,,171-1595568,00.html.

Halprin, D. (2002), *The Expressive Body in Life, Art, and Therapy Working with Movement, Metaphor and Meaning* (London: Jessica Kingsley Publishers).

Hannerz, U. (1990), 'Cosmopolitan and Locals in World Culture', *Theory, Culture & Society* 7, 237–251.

Harrison, G., Hooper, K. and Craig, T. (2001), 'Recovery from psychotic illness: a 15 and 25 year international follow-up study', *British Journal of Psychiatry* 178, 506–517.

Hartley, J. (1992), *TeleOology: Studies in Television* (London: Routledge).

Hasher, L. and Zacks, R. T. (1984), 'Automatic and effortful processes in memory', *J. Exp Psychol Gen* 108, 356–88.

Hay, A. (2003), 'Brazil Votes To Protect Atlantic Rain Forest', www.globalpolicy.org/socecon/envronmt/2003/1205brazilforest.htm accessed 5/11/2005.

Healy, B. and Renouf, N. (2005), 'Contextualised Social Policy: An Australian Perspective', in Ramon, S. and Williams, J. E. (2005), 39–50.

Health e Communication Forum (2006), 'Why Invest in Health Communication?', www.comminit.com/healthecomm/planning.php?showdetails=350.

Health Communication Partnership (2005), www.comminit.com/redirect.cgi? r=http://www.hcpartnership.org/

Health Communication Materials Database Media/Materials Clearing House, www.m-mc.org/mmc_search.php.

Healthology Staff (2005), 'Club Drugs and HIV: Possible New Strain Offers Wake-up Call', www.sexualhealth.com/article.php?Action=read&article_id=415 (accessed 26 September 2005).

Higgins, V. (1999), *Young teenagers and smoking in 1998* (London: Office of National Statistics).

Hillier, D. (1992), 'Into and Out of Africa – Report of the Sir Winston Churchill Travelling Fellowship 1991', unpublished.

Hobson, D. (2003), *Soap Opera* (Oxford: Polity Press).

Holtgrave, D. and Weber, E. U. (1993), 'Dimensions of risk perception for financial and health risks', *Risk Analysis* 13, 553–558.

Horton, D. and Wohl, R. R. (1956), 'Mass communication and para-social interaction',

Psychiatry 19, 215–229.

House of Commons Report (2001), 'Tackling Obesity in England', *Report by the Comptroller and Auditor General HC220 Session 2000-2001* (London: The Stationery Office).

HM Government (2004), *Every Child Matters: Change for Children 2004* (Nottingham: DfES Publications), www.everychildmatters.gov.uk.

Hume, M. (2006), 'Bird Flu and Chicken Little Culture', Spiked Risk 26 February, www.spiked-online.com/Printable/0000000CAF8F.htm (accessed 26 February 2006).

Humphreys, D. (1997), 'Shredheads go mainstream? Snow boarding and alternative youth', *International Review for the Sociology of Sport* 32:2, 300–14.

Institute of Alcohol Studies (IAS) (2005), *Drinking and Driving: IAS Factsheet* (Cambs: IAS).

Institute of Medicine (2003), *Who Will Keep the Public Healthy?* (Washington DC: National Academy Press).

Irwin A. (1999), 'Science and Citizenship', in Scanlon, E., Whitelegg, E. and Yates. S. (eds) *Context and Channels* (London: Routledge).

Jagdeo, T. P., (1990), *Contraceptive prevalence in Saint Lucia, Castries* (St. Lucia: International Planned Parenthood Federation)

Jasper. J. M. (1990), *Nuclear politics: energy and the state in the United States, Sweden and France* (Princeton, NJ: Princeton University Press)

Jeffrey, L. A. (2002), *Sex and Borders: Gender, National Identity and Prostitution Policy in Thailand* (Vancouver: University of British Columbia Press).

Johnson, B. B. and Covello, V. T. (1987), *The social and cultural construction of risk: essays in the selection and perception of risk* (Springer).

Johnson, (2003), 'Case Study: Health an Ecosystem Approach: Mercury Contamination in the Amazon, Reducing Soil Erosion may Provide a Lasting Solution', www.idrc.ca/uploads/user-S/10588088771Ecohealth_Casestudy_03_e.pdf (accessed 12 October 2005).

Joint Health Surveys Unit (JSU) (2001) *Health Survey of England: The Health of Minority Ethnic Groups.*

Jones, E. E., Farina, A., Hastorf, A. H., Markus, H., Miller, D. T., Scott R. A. and French R. de S. (1984), *Social Stigma: The Psychology of Marked Relationships* (New York: W. H. Freeman and Company).

Juon, H., Ensimger, M. and Dobson, K. (2002), 'A longitudinal study of developmental trajectories to young adult cigarette smoking', *Drug and Alcohol Dependence* 66:3, 303–314.

Kahneman, D., Slovic, P., Tversky, A. (eds) (1982), *Judgment under uncertainty: heuristics and biases* (New York: Cambridge University Press).

Kapferer, J.-N. (1990), *Rumors: Uses, Interpretations, and Images* (New Brunswick, NJ: Transaction), 52–58.

Kasperson, R. E., Renn, O., Slovic, P., Brown, H. S., Emel, J., Goble, R., Kasperson, J. X., and Ratick, S. (1988), 'The social amplification of risk: A conceptual framework', *Risk Analysis* 8, 177–187.

Kasperson, R. E, Jhaveri, N. and Kasperon, J. X. (2001), 'Stigma and Social Amplification of Risk: Towards a Framework of Analysis', in Flynn, J., Slovic, P. and Kunreauther, H. (eds) *Risk, Media and Stigma: Understanding Public Challenges to Modern Science and Technology* (London: Earthscan Publications Ltd).

Kellerman, A. L., Rivara, F. P., Rushforth, N. B., Banton, J. G., Reay, D. T., Francisco, J. T., Locci, A. B., Prodzinzki, J., Hackman, B. B., and Somes, G. (1993), 'Gun ownership as a risk factor for homicide in the home', *New England Journal of Medicine* 329:15, 1084–1091.

Kemali, D., Maj, M., Veltro, F., Crepet, P. and Lobrace, S. (1989), 'Sondaggio sulle Opinione degli Italiani nei Riguardi dei Malati de Mente e Dell'Assistenza Psychiatrica', *Revisito Sperimentale Di Freniatria*, Suppl. 5, 1306–1346.

Kopel, D. B. (2000), 'Guns, Gangs and Preschools: Moving beyond conventional solutions to confront juvenile violence', *Barry Law Review* 63 Summer, www.davekopel.com/2A/ LawRev/Guns-Gangs-Preschools.htm#FN;B64.

Kosslyn, S. M. (1988), 'Aspects of a cognitive neuroscience of mental imagery', *Science* 240, 1621–1626.

Kraus, N., Malmfors, T. and Slovic, P. (1992), ‚Intuitive toxicology: Expert and lay judgments of chemical risks', *Risk Analysis* 12, 215–232.

Krimsky, S. and Golding, D. (1992), *Social theories of risk* (Westport, CT: Praeger-Greenwood).

Kroeber, A.. and Kluckhohn, C. (1952), *Culture* (New York: Meridian Books).

Koh, D., Takahashi, K, Lim, Meng-Kin, Imai Teppei, Chia Sin-Eng, Qian Feng, Ng, V and Fones, C. (2005), 'SARS Risk Perception and Preventive Measures', *Singapore and Japan Emerging Infectious Diseases* 11:4.

Kwankam, S. Y. (2004), 'What E-health can Offer', *Bulletin of the World Health Organisation* 82:10, 800–802.

Lader, D. and Goddard, E. (2005), *Smoking Related Behaviours and Attitudes* (UK: National Office of Statistics).

Lader, M. H. (1987), 'Long-term benzodiazepine use and psychological functioning', in Freeman, H. and Rue, Y. (eds), *The Benzodiazepines in Current Clinical Practice* (Royal Society of Medicine Services International Congress and Symposium Series), 55–70.

—— (1991), 'Avoiding long-term use of benzodiazepine drugs', *Prescriber* March, 79–83.

Laing, R. D. (1967), *The Divided Self* (London: Tavistock Publications).

Laurance, J. (2005), 'Flu How Britain Coped in the 1918 Epidemic', *The Independent*, Saturday 22 October 2005.

Lash, S. (1993), 'Reflexive modernisation: the aesthetic dimension', *Theory Culture and Society* 10, 1–23.

—— (2000), 'Risk culture', in Adam, B., Beck, U. and van Loon, J. (eds), *The Risk Society and Beyond* (London, Sage).

Lash, S., Szerszynski, B. and Wynne, B. (eds) (1996), *Risk, Environment and Modernity: towards a new ecology* (London: Sage).

Lash, S. and Urry, J. (1994), *Economies of signs and space* (London: Sage).

Layder, D. (1997), *Modern social theory* (London: UCL Press).

Le Beau, D., Fox, T., Becker, H. and Mufune, P. (1999), *An Anthropological Assessment of Health Risk Behaviour in Northern Namibia* (Windhoek: Ministry of Health and Social Services).

Le Bretton, D. (2004), 'The Anthropology of Adolescent Risk-taking Behaviours', *Body & Society* 10:1, 1–15.

Leff, J. (ed) (1997), *Care in the Community: Illusion or Reality?* (Chichester: Wiley).

Lewis, P. J. (1999), 'The Ibiza Phenomenon', posted on message board, 3 November 1999, www.aber.ac.uk/hypermail/lists/iges-backup/0034.html.

Levo-Henriksson, R. (1994), 'Eyes upon wings - culture in Finnish and U.S. television news', Helsinki: Yleisradio.

Lichtarowicz, A. (2004), 'Obesity epidemic "out of control"', BBC News 31 October 2004 <http://news.bbc.co.uk/2/hi/africa/3969693.stm viewed February 2006>

Linnerooth-Bayer, J. Lofstedt, R. and Sjostedt G. (eds) (2001), *Transboundary Risk Management* (London: Earthscan Publications Ltd), Chapter 8 'Border Crossings', Jeanne X. Kasperson and Roger E. Kasperson.

Loewenstein, G. F., Weber, E. U., Hsee, C. K. and Welch, N. (2001), 'Risk as feelings', *Psychological Bulletin* 127, 267–286.

Lock, S., Reynold, L. and Tansey, E. (1998), *Ashes to Ashes — The history of smoking and health* (Amsterdam: Rodopi).

Loewenstein, G. F., Weber, E. U., Hsee, C. K., Welch, E. (2001), ,Risk as feelings', *Psychological Bulletin* 127, 267–286.

Lovat, T., Parnell, V., Follers, J., Armstrong, D., Jones, J. and Hill, B. (1994), *New Society and Culture: A Student Text* (Wentworth Falls: Social Science Press).

Lupton D. (2005), 'Lay Discourses and beliefs related to food risks: An Australian perspective', *Sociology of Health and Illness* 27:4, 448–467.

MacDonald, W. A. (1994), *Young Driver Research Program: A Review of Information on Young Driver Crashes (CR 128)* (Canberra: Federal Office of Road Safety).

Manderson L. (2001), 'Reducing health risks in resource-poor settings: The relevance of an anthropological perspective', Geneva: World Health Organization, unpublished background paper for The World Health Report 2002.

Manderson, L. and Tye, L. C. (1997), 'Condom use in heterosexual sex: a review of research, 1985-1994', in Sherr, L., Catalan, J. and Hedge, B. (eds), *The impact of AIDS: psychological and social aspects of HIV infection.* (Chur, Switzerland: Harwood Academic Press).

Marcuse, J. (2000), *The ICE Cube – The ICE Report* (Vancouver: DanceArts).

Masquelier, A. (2000), 'Of Headhunters and Cannibals: Migrancy, Labor, and Consumption in the Mawri Imagination', *Cultural Anthropology* 15:1, 84–126.

Matinga, P.U. and Munthali, A. (2001), 'An ethnographic study on malaria in five selected districts in Malawi', final report submitted to UNICEF Malawi, Lilongwe.

Maycock, G. (2002), 'Estimating the effects of age and experience on accident liability using STATS19 data', *Behavioural research in road safety: 12th seminar* (London: Department for Transport), 1–15.

Mayhew, D., Simpson, H. and Pak, A. (2000), *Changes in collision rates among novice drivers during the first months of driving* (Arlington, VA: Institute for Highway Safety).

McCallum, D.B. and Pavlova, M. T. (eds) (1989), *Effective Risk Communication: The Role and Responsibility of Government and Nongovernment Organizations* (New York: Plenum Press), 45–49.

McCormack, C. (1994), 'The Health Promotion Gap', *Healthlines* 13, 10.

McDaniels, T. and Gregory, R. (1991), *A framework for structuring cross-cultural research on risk and decision making*, *Journal of Cross-Cultural Psychology* 22, 103–128.

McFadden, P. (ed) (1992), 'Sex, Sexuality and the Problem of AIDS in Africa', in Meena, R., *Gender in Southern Africa: Conceptual and Theoretical Issues* (Harare: SAPES Books).

McGuire, W. J. (1984), 'Public Communication as a Strategy for Inducing Health-Promoting Behavioral Change', *Preventive Medicine* 13:3, 299–313.

McLuhan, M.(1964), *Understanding Media* (London: Routledge).

McPherson, B., Curtis, J. and Loy, J. (1989), *The Social Significance of Sport: An Introduction to the Sociology of Sport* (Champaign: Human Kinetics Books).

Mezzina, R. (2005), 'Paradigm Shift in Psychiatry: Processes and Outcomes', in Ramon, S. and Williams, J. E. (2005), 81–94.

Mills, K. (2003), *Smokescreen* (London: Hodder & Stoughton).

Mitchell, R. C. and Carson, R. T. (1989), *Using surveys to value public goods: the contingent valuation method* (Washington, DC: Resources for the Future).

Morgan, M. G., Fischhoff, B., Bostrom, A., and Atman, C. J. (2002), *Risk communication: A mental models approach* (New York: Cambridge University Press).

Mosher, L. and Burti, L. (1989), *Community Mental Health: Principles and Practice* (London: W.W. Norton).

Munthali, A. C. (2005), 'Managing Malaria in Under-Five Children in a Rural Malawian Village', *Nordic Journal of African Studies* 14:2, 127–146.

Narasimham, M. V. V. L. (1991), Proceedings of an Informal Consultative Meeting (eds Sharma, V. P. and Kondrashin, A. V.), 81–91.

National Research Council (1989), *Improving Risk Communication* (Washington, D.C.: National Academy Press).

Newman, M. L., Holden, G.W. and Delville, Y. (2005), 'Isolation and the stress of being bullied', *Journal of Adolescence* 28: 343–357.

New York City Department of Health (2000), *Comprehensive Arthropod-borne Disease Surveillance and Control Plan 2000* (New York, NY; DoH).

Nevid, J. (2000), 'Smoking Cessation and Ethnic Minorities: Fighting Back Against Joe Camel', www.vincenter.org/96/nevid.html.

Otway, H. and Wynne, B. (1989), 'Risk communication: Paradigm and paradox', *Risk Analysis* 9:2, 141–146.

Palmara, P. and Stevenson, M. (2003), 'A longitudinal investigation of psychosocial risk factors for speeding offences among young motor car drivers', Report No. RR128 (Univ. Western Australia).

Palmer, C. (1999), 'Smells like extreme spirit: Punk music, skate culture and the packaging of extreme sports', in Bloustien, G. (ed.) 'Musical Visions', selected conference proceedings from 6th National Australian/New Zealand IASPM and Inaugural Arnhem Land Performance Conference (Adelaide: Wakefield Press).

—— (2002), '"Shit happens": the selling of risk in extreme sport - Interlaken and Everest tourist tragedies', *Australian Journal of Anthropology*, December, www.findarticles.com/p/articles/mi_m2472/is_3_13/ai_95148966.

Papa, M. J., Singhal, A., Law, S., Sood, S., Rogers, E.M. and Shefner-Rogers, C. L. (2000), 'Entertainment-education and social change: An analysis of parasocial interaction, social learning, collective efficacy, and paradoxical communication', *Journal of Communication* 50:4, 31–55.

Pascal, B. (1910), *Pascal's Pensées*, translated by W. F. Trotter (composed in 1600s, first published in 1800s), Pensees section 343, (Penguin).

Pelto, P. J. and Pelto, G. H. (1997), 'Studying knowledge, culture and behaviour in applied medical anthropology', *Medical Anthropology Quarterly* 11, 147–63.

Peters, E. and Slovic, P. (1996), 'The role of affect and worldviews as orienting dispositions in the perception and acceptance of nuclear power', *Journal of Applied Social Psychology* 26, 1427–53.

Peterson, C. R. and Beach, L.R. (1967), 'Man as an intuitive statistician', *Psychol Bull* 69, 29–46.

Philo, G. (ed) (1996), *The Media and Mental Distress* (London: Longman).

Pidgeon, N. F., Hood, C., Jones, D., Turner, B. and Gibson, R. (1992), 'Risk perception'. Ch. 5 of *Risk - Analysis, Perception and Management: Report of a Royal Society Study Group* (London, The Royal Society), 89–134.

Piotrow, P. T., Rimon, J. G., Payne Merritt, A.. and Saffittz, G. (2003), *Advancing Health Communication: The PCS Experience in the Field*, Center Publication 103 (Baltimore: Johns Hopkins Bloomberg School of Public Health/Center for Communications Programs).

Population Communications International (PCI) (2006), 'Telling Stories Saving Lives', www.population.org/aboutpci.shtml (accessed February 2006).

Population Reference Bureau (PRB) (1997), *World Population Data Sheet* (Washington, DC: PRB).

—— (2000), *World Population Data Sheet* (Washington, DC: PRB).

Porter, K. A. (1990) (originally written in 1939), *Pale Horse, Pale Rider* (Orlando, Fla.:Harcourt Brace Jovanavich).

Proctor, R. (1999), *The Nazi War on Cancer* (Princeton: Princeton University Press).

Prochaska, J. O. and Di Clemente, C. C. (1982), 'Transtheoretical therapy: toward a more integrative model of change', *Psychotherapy: Theory, Research, Practice* 19, 276–88.

Prochaska, J. O. and Velicer, W. F. (1997), 'The transtheoretical model of health behavior change', *American Journal of Health Promotion* 12, 38–48.

Prochaska, J. O., Redding, C. A. and Evers, K. E. (1997), 'The transtheoretical model and stages of change', in Glanz, K., Lewis, F. & Rimer B. (eds), *Health behavior and health education: Theory, research, and practice* 2nd edn (San Francisco, CA: Jossey-Bass), 60–84.

Rahman, M. M., Sengupta, M. K., Ahamed, S., Chowdhury, U. K., Lodh, D., Hossain, A., Das, B., Roy, N., Saha, K.C., Palit, S. K., Chakraborti, D. (2005), 'Arsenic Contamination of groundwater and its health impact on residents in a village in West Bengal, India', *Bulletin of the World Health Organisation* 83:1, 49–57.

Ramon, S. (ed.) (1990), *Psychiatry in Transition: British and Italian Approaches* (London: Pluto Press).

—— (ed.) (2000), *A Stakeholder's Approach to Innovation in Mental Health: A Reader for the 21st Century* (Brighton: Pavilion Publishing).

—— (2005), 'Approaches to Risk in Mental Health: A Multidisciplinary Discourse', in Tew, J. (ed.) *Social Perspectives in Mental Health: Developing Social Models to Understand and Work with Mental Distress* (London: Jessica Kingsley Publishers).

Ramon, S. and Savio, M. (2000), 'A Scandal of the 80s and 90s: Media Representations of Mental Illness Issues in Britain and Italy', in Ramon, S. (2000).

Ramon, S. and Williams, J. E. (eds) (2005), *Mental Health at the Crossroad: The Promise of the Psychosocial Approach* (Aldershot: Ashgate Publishing).

Rapaport, J. (2005), 'The Informal Caring Experience: Issues and Dilemmas' in Ramon, S. and Williams, J. E. (2005), 155–170.

Rasmussen, S., Prescott, E., Sørensen, T. and Søgaard, J. (2004), 'The total lifetime costs of smoking', *The European Journal of Public Health* 14:1, 95–100.

Regis, A. and Butler, P. (1997), *RESPONSIBILITY 6: Researching and evaluating St. Lucia's population "problem" offers new solutions in broadcasting on lifestyle issues for today's youth* (Castries, St. Lucia: RARE Center).

Registrar of Civil Status and Statistics Department (1994), *Census, Volume 3: Living Arrangements and Fertility 1991* (Castries, St. Lucia: Government of St. Lucia).

Repper, J. and Perkins, R. (2003), *Social Inclusion and Recovery: A Model for Mental Health Practice* (Edinburgh: Balliere Tindall).

Reynolds, B. and Seeger, M. W. (2005), 'Crisis and Emergency Risk Communication as an Integrative Model', Journal of Health Communication e-newsletter, May 2005; *Journal of Health Communication* 10, 43–55.

Riddle, M. (2005), 'The Madness in Our Midst: Far from Imprisoning Too Few, We are Continuing to Lock Up Too Many', *The Observer*, 20 March, p. 28.

Rinehart, R. (1998a), *Players All: Performance in Contemporary Sport* (Bloomington: Indiana University Press).

—— (1998b), 'Inside of the outside: Pecking orders within alternative sport at ESPN's 1995 "The eXtreme Games"', *Journal of Sport and Social Issues* 22:4, 398–415.

Roberts, G. and Wolfson, P. (2004), 'The Rediscovery of Recovery: Open to All', *Advances in Psychiatry* 10, 37–49.

Robertson, R. (1992), *Globalization: Social Theory and Global Culture* (London: Sage).

Romanyshyn, R. D. and Whalen, B. J. (1987), 'Depression and the American dream. The struggle with home', in Levin, D. M. (ed.), *Pathologies of the modern self. Postmodern studies in narcissism, schizophrenia, and depression* (New York: New York University Press), 198–220.

Roos, P. A. (1985), *Gender and Work* (Albany, NY: State University of New York Press).

Rottenstreich, Y. and Hsee, C. K. (2001), 'Money, kisses and electric shocks: On the affective psychology of probability weighting', *Psychological Science* 12:3, 185–90.

Royal College of Physicians (2000), *Nicotine Addiction in Britain* (London: RCP).

Rubin, A. M. and Perse, E. M. (1987), 'Audience activity and soap opera involvement: A uses and effects investigation', *Human Communication Research* 14, 246–268.

Saba, W. (2006), Response to question on Health e- communication discussion groups 11 February 2006 <http://forums.comminit.com/viewtopic.php?p=145969&style=1#145969>

Sabo, D. and Gordon, D. (1995), *Men's Health and Illness: Gender, Power and the Body* (London: Sage).

Sandman P. M. (1989), 'Hazard versus outrage in the public perception of risk', in Covello, V. T., McCallum, D.B. and Pavlova, M.T. (eds) (1989), 45–49.

Sandman, P. (2001), 'Anthrax, Bioterrorism, and Risk Communication: Guidelines for Action', www.psandman.com/col/part2.htm.

Sandman, P. (2002), 'Smallpox Vaccination: Some Risk Communication Linchpins', www.psandman.com/col/smallpox.htm.

Scheff, T. (1975, 1999), *Being Mentally Ill: A Sociological Theory* (New York: Aldine de Gruyter).

Schwartz, S. H. (1992), 'Universals in the content and structure of values: Theoretical advances and empirical tests in 20 countries', in M. P. Zanna (ed.), *Advances in experimental social psychology* Vol. 25 (Orlando: Academic Press), 1–65.

Shafey, O., Dolwick, S. and Guindon, G. (eds) (2003), *Tobacco Country Profiles* (American Cancer Society/WHO/International Union Against Cancer).

Silagy, C., Lancaster, T., Stead, L., Mant, D., Fowler, G. (2004), 'Nicotine replacement therapy for smoking cessation', *The Cochrane Database of Systematic Reviews 2004*, Issue 3.

Simons-Morton, G. (2003), *The protective effect of parental expectations against early adolescent smoking initiation: Health Education Research*, doi:10.1093/her/cyg071 (Oxford University Press).

Simons-Morton, B. (2004), 'The protective effect of parental expectations against early adolescent smoking initiation', *Health Education Research* 19:1, 561–569.

Singapore Health Promotion Board , www.hpb.gov.sg/hpb/default.asp?pg id=985.

Singhal, A. (2003), 'Overview and Executive Summary of the Taru Project Qualitative Report',

Population Communications International , www.population.org/multimedia/Taru-Qual-reports-exec-summary1.pdf (accessed January 2006).

—— (2004), 'Entertainment education through participatory theater: Freirean strategies for empowering the oppressed', in A. Singhal, M. Cody, E. M. Rogers and M. Sabido (eds), *Entertainment-education and social change: History, research, and practice* (Mahwah, NJ: Lawrence Erlbaum).

Singh, N., Singh, M. P., Saxena, A., Sharma, V. P. and Kalra, N. L. (1998), 'Knowledge, attitude, beliefs and practices (KABP) study related to malaria and intervention strategies in ethnic tribals of Mandla (Madhya Pradesh)', www.iisc.ernet.in/~currsci/dec25/articles25.htm.

Sloman, S. A. (1996), 'The empirical case for two systems of reasoning', *Psychological Bulletin* 119:1, 3–22.

Slovic, P. (1987), 'Perception of risk', *Science* 236, 280–285.

—— (1992), 'Perception of risk: Reflections on the psychometric paradigm', in S. Krimsky and D. Golding (eds), *Social theories of risk* (New York: Praeger), 117–152.

—— (1999), 'Trust, emotion, sex, politics, and science: Surveying the risk-assessment battlefield', *Risk Analysis*, 19:4, 689–701. Originally published in M. H. Bazerman, D. M. Messick, A. E. Tenbrunsel and K. A. Wade-Benzoni (eds) (1997), *Environment, ethics, and behavior* (San Francisco: New Lexington), 277–313. Revised version in *The University of Chicago Legal Forum*, 1997, 59–99.

—— (2000), *The Perception of Risk* (London: Earthscan).

—— (2002), 'Terrorism as hazard: A new species of trouble', *Risk Analysis* 22:3, 425–6.

Slovic, P., Finucane, M., Peters, E. and MacGregor, D. G. (2002), 'The affect heuristic', in T. Gilovich, D. Griffin, and D. Kahneman (eds), *Heuristics and biases: the psychology of intuitive judgment* (New York: Cambridge University Press), 397–420.

Slovic, P., Fischhoff, B., Lichtenstein, S. (1979), 'Rating the risks', *Environment* 21, 14–20, 36–9.

—— (1984), 'Behavioral decision theory perspectives on risk and safety', *Acta Psychologica* 56, 183–203.

Slovic, P., Malmfors, T., Mertz, C. K., Neil, N. and Purchase, I. F. (1997), 'Evaluating chemical risks: results of a survey of the British Toxicology Society', *Human and Experimental Toxicology* 16, 289–304.

Smith, K. R., Corvalan, C. F., and Kjellstrom, T. (1999), 'How much global ill health is attributable to environmental factors?', *Epidemiology* 10:5, 573–584.

Snow, P. and Bruce, D. (2003), 'Cigarette smoking in teenage girls: exploring the role of peer reputations, self-concept and coping', *Health Education Research* 18:4, 439–452.

Snowden, A., Arblaster, L. and Stead, L. (2003), 'Community interventions for preventing smoking in young people', *Cochrane Database of Systematic Reviews* 1.

Sofoulis, Z. (2003), 'Driving Scenarios in Australian Car Advertising', *RoundAbout: Mobility, Narratives and Journeys in 20th Century Australia Conference* (History Department, Sydney University).

Sofoulis, Z., Noble, G. and Redshaw, S. (2005), 'Transforming Drivers: Driving as Social, Cultural and Gendered Practice', University of Western Sydney and National Roads and Motorists' Association Limited (NRMA Motoring and Services), www.mynrma.com.au/files/1/Transforming%20drivers.pdf.

Sood, S. and Rogers, E. M. (2000), 'Dimensions of parasocial interaction by letterwriters to a popular entertainment-education soap opera in India', *Journal of Broadcasting and Electronic Media* 44:3, 389–414.

Statistics Department (1993), *Vital Statistics Report, 1992* (Castries, St. Lucia: Government of St. Lucia).

—— (1994), *Vital Statistics Report, 1993* (Castries, St. Lucia: Government of St. Lucia).

Stevens, A. and Caan, W. (forthcoming), 'Gender, economics and culture: diversity and the international evolution of tobacco consumption' (submitted to *Tobacco Control*).

Stoler, A. L. (2002), *Carnal knowledge and imperial power: race and the intimate in colonial rule* (Berkeley: University of California Press).

Swinburn, B., Gill, T. and Kumanyika, S. (2005), 'Obesity Prevention: A proposal framework for Translating Evidence into Action', *Obesity Review* 6, 23–33.

Talavera, P. (2002), *Challenging the Namibian perception of sexuality: A case study of the Ovahima and Ovaherero culturo-sexual models in Kunene North in the HIV/AIDS context* (Windhoek: Gamsberg MacMillan Publishers (Pty) Ltd).

Taussig, M. (1987), *Shamanism, Colonialism, and the Wild Man: A Study in Terror and Healing* (Chicago: University of Chicago Press).

Taylor, P. J. and Gunn, A. (1999), 'Homicides by people with mental illness: myth and reality', *British Journal of Psychiatry* 174, 9–14.

Thomas, R. (2002), 'School-based programmes for preventing smoking', *Cochrane Database of Systematic Reviews* 2.

Thompson, M. (1992), 'The dynamics of cultural theory and their implications for the enterprise culture', in S. Hargreaves-Heap and A. Ross (eds), *Understanding the Enterprise Culture* (Edinburgh: Edinburgh University Press), 182–202.

Tibinyane, N. (2003), 'Are Reproductive Rights Respected and Promoted in Namibia?', *The Namibian*, 9 December 2003.

Tinkler, P. (2003), 'Refinement & Respectable Consumption: the Acceptable Face of Women's Smoking in Britain, 1913–1970', *Gender & History* 15:2, 342–360.

Treichler, P. (1999). 'AIDS and HIV Infection in the Third World: A First World Chronicle', in Treichler, P. A., *How to Have Theory in an Epidemic. Cultural Chronicles of AIDS* (Durham: Duke University Press), 99–126.

Triandis, H. C. (1989), 'Cross-Cultural Studies of Individualism and Collectivism', in J. Berman (ed.), *Nebraska Symposium* (Lincoln, NE: University of Nebraska Press), 41–130.

Tulloch, J. and Lupton, D. (1997), *Television, AIDS and Risk: A cultural studies approach to health communication* (New South Wales, Australia: Allen and Unwin).

Turner, V. (1969), *The Ritual Process: Structure and Anti-Structure* (Chicago: Aldine Publishing Company).

Turner, C. and McClure, R. (2003), 'Age and gender differences in risk-taking behaviour as an explanation for high incidence of motor vehicle crashes as a driver in young males', *Injury Control and Safety Promotion* 10:3, 123–130.

Tversky, A. and Kahneman, D. (1973), 'Availability: A heuristic for judging frequency and probability', *Cognitive Psychology* 5, 207–232.

Tversky, A. and Kahneman, D. (1974), 'Judgment under uncertainty: Heuristics and biases', *Science* 185, 1124–1131.

UNICEF (2005), *The State Of The World's Children Report: Childhood under threat* (New York: UNICEF).

United Nations (1997), *Kyoto Protocol To The United Nations Framework Convention On Climate Change* (New York: United Nations).

—— (2002), *HIV/AIDS Awareness and Behaviour* (New York. United Nations).

United Nations Secretariat (2002a), *HIV/AIDS: Awareness and Behaviour-Executive Summary* (New York: United Nations).

—— (2002b), *HIV/AIDS and Fertility in Sub-Saharan Africa: A Review of the Research Literature* (New York: United Nations).

Van Gennep (1960), *The Rites of Passage* (Chicago: University of Chicago Press).

Vaughan, P. W., Regis A. and St. Catherine, E. (2000), 'Effects of an Entertainment-Education Radio Soap Opera on Family Planning And HIV Prevention in St. Lucia', *International Family Planning Perspectives* 26:4, 148–157.

von Winterfeld, D. and Edwards, W. (1984), 'Patterns of conflict about risky technologies', *Risk Analysis* 4, 55–68.

Wade-Benzoni, K. A., Tenbrunsel, A. E., and Bazerman, M. H. (1996), 'Egocentric Interpretations of Fairness in Asymmetric, Environmental Social Dilemmas: Explaining Harvesting Behavior and the Role of Communication', *Organizational Behavior and Human Decision Processes* 67, 111–126. Cited in Bazerman, M. H. and Watkins, M. D. (2004).

Warner, R. (1985 and 1994), *Recovery from Schizophrenia* (London: Routledge).

Waters, M. (1995), *Globalization* (London: Routledge).

Watson, J. (1998), 'Running around like a lunatic: Colin's body and the case of male embodiment', in S. Nettleton and J. Watson (eds), *The body in everyday life* (London: Routledge), 163–79.

Web, G. P. (2002) *Nutrition: A health promotion approach* (2nd Ed). London: Hodder Arnold

Weber, E. U. (1997), 'Perception and expectation of climate change: Precondition for economic and technological adaptation', in M. Bazerman, D. Messick, A. Tenbrunsel and K. Wade-Benzoni (eds), *Psychological Perspectives to Environmental and Ethical Issues in Management* (San Francisco, CA: Jossey-Bass), 314–341.

—— (2001a), 'Personality and risk taking', in N. J. Smelser and P. B. Baltes (eds), *International Encyclopedia of the Social and Behavioral Sciences* (Oxford, UK: Elsevier Science Limited), 11274–11276.

—— (2001b), 'Decision and choice: Risk, empirical studies', in N. J. Smelser and P. B. Baltes (eds), *International Encyclopedia of the Social and Behavioral Sciences* (Oxford, UK: Elsevier Science Limited), 13347–13351.

Weber, E. U., Blais, A.-R. and Betz, N. (2002), 'A domain-specific risk-attitude scale: Measuring risk perceptions and risk behaviors', *Journal of Behavioral Decision Making*, 15, 1–28.

Weber, E. U. and Hsee, C. K. (1998), 'Cross-cultural differences in risk perception but cross-cultural similarities in attitudes towards risk', *Management Science*, 44, 1205–1217.

—— (1999), 'Models and mosaics: Investigating cross-cultural differences in risk perception and risk preference', *Psychonomic Bulletin & Review*, 6, 611–617.

Weber, E. U. and Milliman, R. (1997), 'Perceived risk attitudes: Relating risk perception to risky choice', *Management Science* 43, 122–143.

Weber, E. U., Sharoni, S. and Blais, A.-R. (2001), 'Predicting risk-sensitivity in humans and lower animals: Risk as variance or coefficient of variation', *Psychological Review*, forthcoming.

Weinstein, N. D. and Sandman, P. M. (1992), 'A Model of the Precaution Adoption Process: Evidence From Home Radon Testing', *Health Psychology* 11:3, 170–180.

Whitburn, V. (1999), 'Archers star launches Rwanda soap', 16 Feb 1999 <http://news.bbc.co.uk/1/hi/entertainment/270427.stm>

Wilde, G. J. S. (1994), *Target risk: Dealing with the danger of death, disease and damage in everyday decisions* (Ontario, Canada: PDE Publications).

Wilde G. (1998), 'Risk homeostasis theory: an overview', *Injury Prevention* 4, 89–91.

Williams, A. (2000), 'Graduated licensing in the United States', Proceedings of the *65th Road Safety Congress* (Plymouth: Royal Society for the Prevention of Accidents).

World Health Organization (WHO) (1997), 'Obesity: Preventing and Managing the Global Epidemic', *Report of a WHO Consultation on Obesity, Geneva, 3–5 June*.

—— (2002), *World Report on Violence and Health, Geneva, October*, www.who.int/violence_injury_prevention/main.cfm?p=0000000117.

—— (2003), *Mobilizing for Action, Communication for Behavioral Impact (COMBI)* (Tunis: Mediterranean Center for Vulnerability Reduction).

Wyer, Robert S., Jr., and Thomas Srull (1986), "Human Cognition in Its Social Context," Psychological Review 93 (July), 322-359.

Wynne, B. (1992), 'Risk and social learning: Reification to engagement', in S. Krimsky and D. Golding (eds), *Social theories of risk* (Westport, CT: Praeger), 275–300.

Yang, G., Ma J., Chen. A., Brown, S., Taylor. C. and Samet. J. (2004), 'Smoking among adolescents in China: 1998 survey findings', *International Journal of Epidemiology* 33:5, 1103–1110.

Zaim, M., Nejad-Naseeri, D., Azoordegan, F. and Emadi, A. M. (1997), 'Knowledge and practice of residents about malaria in southeast Iran (1994)', *Acta Tropica* 64, 123–130.

Zipes, J. (1986), *Don't Bet on the Prince: Contemporary Feminist Fairy Tales in North America and England* (New York: Methuen).

Index

Join our e-mail newsletter

Gower is widely recognized as one of the world's leading publishers on management and business practice. Its programmes range from 1000-page handbooks through practical manuals to popular paperbacks. These cover all the main functions of management: human resource development, sales and marketing, project management, finance etc. Gower also produces training videos and activities manuals on a wide range of management skills.

As our list is constantly developing you may find it difficult to keep abreast of new titles. With this in mind we offer a free e-mail news service, approximately once every two months, which provides a brief overview of the most recent titles and links to our catelogue, should you wish to read more or see sample pages.

To sign up to this service, send your request via e-mail to info@gowerpub.com. Please put your e-mail address in the body of the e-mail as confirmation of your agreement to receive information in this way.

GOWER